Eating Behavior and Obesity

Behavioral Economics Strategies for Health Professionals

T0211372

Shahram Heshmat, PhD, is an Associate Professor of Public Health and Economics at the University of Illinois at Springfield and an Adjunct Associate Professor of Medical Humanities at Southern Illinois University. His research is aimed at understanding the role of emotions in consumer behavior and well-being, applications of the principles of behavioral economics to appetitive behavior, changing health behavior, and designing prevention policies.

Eating Behavior and Obesity

Behavioral Economics Strategies
for Health Professionals

Shahram Heshmat, PhD

SPRINGER PUBLISHING COMPANY
NEW YORK

Springer Publishing Company, LLC
11 West 42nd Street
New York, NY 10036
www.springerpub.com

Acquisitions Editor: Jennifer Perillo
Senior Editor: Rose Mary Piscitelli
Composition: S4Carlisle Publishing Services

ISBN: 978-0-8261-0621-6
E-book ISBN: 978-0-8261-0622-3

11 12 13/ 5 4 3 2 1

The author and the publisher of this Work have made every effort to use sources believed to be reliable to provide information that is accurate and compatible with the standards generally accepted at the time of publication. The author and publisher shall not be liable for any special, consequential, or exemplary damages resulting, in whole or in part, from the readers' use of, or reliance on, the information contained in this book. The publisher has no responsibility for the persistence or accuracy of URLs for external or third-party Internet Web sites referred to in this publication and does not guarantee that any content on such Web sites is, or will remain, accurate or appropriate.

Library of Congress Cataloging-in-Publication Data
Heshmat, Shahram.
    Eating behavior and obesity / Shahram Heshmat.
        p. cm.
    Includes bibliographical references.
    ISBN 978-0-8261-0621-6 — ISBN 978-0-8261-0622-3 (E-book)
    1. Eating disorders.   2. Decision making—Psychological aspects.   I. Title
    [DNLM: 1. Eating Disorders.   2. Feeding Behavior—psychology.   3. Decision Making.   4. Obesity.
    5. Socioeconomic Factors. WM 175]
    RC685.A65H47 2011
    616.85'26—dc23   2011017984

Special discounts on bulk quantities of our books are available to corporations, professional associations, pharmaceutical companies, health care organizations, and other qualifying groups.

If you are interested in a custom book, including chapters from more than one of our titles, we can provide that service as well.

For details, please contact:
Special Sales Department, Springer Publishing Company, LLC
11 West 42nd Street, 15th Floor, New York, NY 10036-8002
Phone: 877-687-7476 or 212-431-4370; Fax: 212-941-7842
Email: sales@springerpub.com

Printed in the United States of America by Gasch Printing

Springer Publishing Company, LLC
11 West 42nd Street
New York, NY 10036
www.springerpub.com

Acquisitions Editor: Jennifer Perillo
Senior Editor: Rose Mary Piscitelli
Composition: S4Carlisle Publishing Services

ISBN: 978-0-8261-0621-6
E-book ISBN: 978-0-8261-0622-3

11 12 13/ 5 4 3 2 1

The author and the publisher of this Work have made every effort to use sources believed to be reliable to provide information that is accurate and compatible with the standards generally accepted at the time of publication. The author and publisher shall not be liable for any special, consequential, or exemplary damages resulting, in whole or in part, from the readers' use of, or reliance on, the information contained in this book. The publisher has no responsibility for the persistence or accuracy of URLs for external or third-party Internet Web sites referred to in this publication and does not guarantee that any content on such Web sites is, or will remain, accurate or appropriate.

Library of Congress Cataloging-in-Publication Data
Heshmat, Shahram.
  Eating behavior and obesity / Shahram Heshmat.
     p. cm.
  Includes bibliographical references.
  ISBN 978-0-8261-0621-6 — ISBN 978-0-8261-0622-3 (E-book)
  1. Eating disorders. 2. Decision making—Psychological aspects. I. Title
  [DNLM: 1. Eating Disorders. 2. Feeding Behavior—psychology. 3. Decision Making. 4. Obesity.
  5. Socioeconomic Factors. WM 175]
  RC685.A65H47 2011
  616.85′26—dc23   2011017984

Printed in the United States of America by Gasch Printing

Eating Behavior and Obesity

Behavioral Economics Strategies
for Health Professionals

Shahram Heshmat, PhD

SPRINGER PUBLISHING COMPANY
NEW YORK

Contents

Preface

This book utilizes *behavioral economics* as the overarching conceptual framework to discuss the root causes of obesity. This relatively new field blends insights from psychology and economics. Behavioral economics is a generalization of *rational choice theory*, which incorporates concepts of rationality, willpower, and self-interest in a systemic way. Its basic premise is that humans are hardwired to make judgment errors and they need a "nudge" to make decisions that are in their own best interest. The field of behavioral economics is mostly unknown to practitioners in public health, yet it can offer a valuable framework for understanding health behavior for public health professionals. Principles of behavioral economics can capture the complexity of individual judgments and health behaviors; this makes it a useful foundation for improving health promotion policy.

Behavioral economics provides a framework to understand when and how people make errors. Basic tenets of behavioral economics demonstrate that the environment plays an important role in eating and body weight regulation. This introductory text integrates the basic concepts of behavioral economics and public health to increase our understanding of individual eating behaviors that can then be integrated into the formulation of preventive strategies.

The traditional economic perspective relies on a "market" approach, in which individuals are assumed to be making autonomous decisions based on their own preferences with a goal of maximizing individual satisfaction. However, many of these assumptions are inaccurate and simply do not fit what we know about individual behavior from public health. Human beings have limited cognitive abilities and limited willpower. Conscious and unconscious factors influence people's decisions in ways that cause us to act against our own best interest. As will be discussed throughout this text, biases, gut feelings, and habits often compete with deliberate consideration of information. While individuals may be aware of the factors that contribute to obesity, their everyday lifestyle choices do not reflect this knowledge. Rather, these choices are often made in an unconscious and more impulsive manner. Because of this, individuals frequently make decisions that depart systematically from the predictions of economists' standard rational model. Behavioral economics attempts to understand these departures and, more generally, integrate psychologists' understanding of human behavior into economic analysis. Identifying ways in which behavior systematically deviates from optimality can then generate new insights into the underlying choice mechanism. Understanding why, how, and when people choose certain foods and consume them in certain amounts is a useful approach to preventing or simply changing potentially unhealthy eating behavior that contributes to obesity. Based on the findings and methods of behavioral economics, the book presents intervention strategies to help individuals to improve their eating behavior and enhance their well-being. Armed with the information presented in this text, it is hoped that readers understand the psychology behind excessive eating and learn how to promote a long-term healthy lifestyle.

OBJECTIVE

The purpose of this book is to present a behavioral economics perspective on food choice. An understanding of the factors that influence food choice helps reveal some of the difficulties, as well as solutions, in directing individuals toward healthier eating behavior. From a behavioral economics perspective, public policy attempts to foster healthy eating behaviors that focus on understanding and changing the way individuals make food decisions.

Behavioral economics identifies a large number of circumstances in which people seem to behave inconsistently and in which their decisions deviate from what is predicted by the rational principles of the standard economic model. Identifying these conditions provides an understanding of, for example, what factors make it harder for dieters to resist attractive food, and will help dieters to resist temptation. Knowing why people fail to maintain a desired healthy behavior over time will go some ways toward avoiding relapse, and to move people in a direction that will make their lives better.

It is hoped that this book will enhance the understanding of decision-making processes that underlie maintaining a desired healthy behavior over the long term. This is accomplished by looking at conditions in which the decision making is impaired or even breaks down. The knowledge of these biases should help dieters to develop problem-solving skills in weight management. A recent review of studies on the effectiveness of economics concepts to better understand the barriers to making healthy choices by individuals. This book would be useful as a stand-alone or as a supplementary book in courses such as health economics, health behavior, and public health policy. The book does not assume advanced knowledge of economics or decision analysis.

Preparing this book has been a quite challenging and enriching experience for me. I have learned a great deal. Moreover, the experience has changed the way I think and behave with regard to food. I hope that similar benefits will be passed to you, the reader, as well.

Acknowledgments

The study of behavioral economics of food choice has been at the center of my research and teaching over the past 5 years. The work presented here is a reflection of countless influences. Several authors have shaped my views on this topic: Ainslie, Damasio, Elster, Kahneman, Loewenstein, Wansink, and many others. I am deeply grateful to all those who have contributed to the development of my perspective.

The initial preparation of this book took place while I taught a course in the Department of Public Health at the University of Illinois at Springfield. I have gained a great deal of insights and feedback from students as I struggled to explain my understanding of the relevance of behavioral economics to eating behavior.

I am also grateful to those who have supported my effort in completing this project. These include my beloved wife, Monica, whose patience and sensitivity have been a great support, as well as my two children, Colin and Claire. I am very grateful to my family for tolerating me while I struggled to prepare this book. Finally, I owe special thanks to my editor, Jennifer Perillo, for her support and encouragement in developing this book. Her refusal to tolerate my inclination to procrastinate gave me a powerful incentive to complete it on time. I regret any errors that may appear in this book and take full responsibility for them.

1

Behavioral Economics and Eating Decisions

INTRODUCTION

Individual lifestyle choices are fundamental to improvements in health status. About half of all deaths in the United States are attributable to a small number of preventable behaviors and exposures, such as smoking, poor diet, and lack of exercise.[1] Next to smoking, obesity is the leading behavioral cause of death. With the decline in the prevalence of smoking, obesity may have become the most important determinants of health. People who maintain nutritious diets lower their risk of certain diseases. There is an increasing awareness that dietary intervention can prevent, delay, and treat many common diseases and enhance the quality and length of life. As a consequence of the rising cost of conventional medical treatment and drugs, health-care providers and public health policy makers are increasingly looking to diet as a means to decrease the incidence of many chronic and age-related diseases.

Dieting, a conscious restriction of food intake to prevent weight gain or promote weight loss, is a popular means of weight control. Americans spend many billions of dollars each year trying to lose weight through dieting and/or exercise. Estimates are that about half of men and two-thirds of women are trying to lose weight at any given time (Sreoebe, 2008). Despite documented short-term success, most diet plans have very low success rates, and most dieters regain their weight back within 3–5 years[2] (Hill, 1999; IOM, 2003). About half the people on weight loss programs are likely to weigh more 4 years after their diet than they did before (Mann et al., 2007). This indicates that dieters are eating more than their bodies need to maintain energy balance.[3] Dieters tend to display disinhibited

---

[1]According to the American Cancer Society, about a third of the 550,000 American cancer deaths each year are linked to obesity, poor diet, and inactivity. Another third are due to smoking.

[2]People facing serious illness such as heart attack or stroke are three times more likely to quit smoking than lose weight. One reason for the disparity is the lack of insurance coverage for weight-loss programs (Keenan, 2009).

[3]The limited success of dieting may be due to an incomplete understanding of the factors that increase risk of obesity.

eating in response to a wide variety of events. These events disrupt self-control and often trigger episodic overeating that wipes out all the dietary achievements made since the last overeating episode.

The observation that initial dieting and weight loss success does not ensure continued success suggests that greater attention must be given to the factors that underlie dieters' decision to maintain a pattern of successful diet behavior (Rothman, 2000, 2004). Why is it that people who are able to successfully initiate changes in their behavior have difficulty maintaining it over time? One possible answer is that people have self-control problems in the form of a *present-biased preference*. Present bias is normally expressed as a self-control problem, where one places extra value on a more immediate reward than a longer term reward. Present bias is viewed as an "error." That is, it is a bias that can lead people not to behave in their own best interests. Our short-term inclinations about what to do often do not accord with our own assessment of what is in our long-term best interests—maintaining healthy diets. In general, present bias explains why many behaviors that undermine health involve immediate benefits (such as overeating) coupled with delayed costs (such as obesity). For example, present bias explains individuals' poor decision making behind smoking and other preventable conditions, which contribute to 40% of premature deaths (McGinnis, 1999). Many preventable diseases and premature deaths could be prevented if we change people's present-oriented behavior, par-ticularly with regard to overeating.

DETERMINANTS OF FOOD CHOICE

This book is essentially about consumer behavior in the context of food choice; it aims to increase understanding of why we eat and how much we eat. Given that food choice is a product of both environmen-tal and biological interactions, a full understanding of eating behavior should include both the internal biological signals and external environ-ment contributing to food intake. One must also understand the role of irrational forces as well as rational causes of obesity. Behavioral econom-ics demonstrates how flawed decisions and self-control problems can impact eating behavior. So we need to explore ways to improve decision making and health habits in order to improve health.

In general, eating behavior can be modeled as including four stages: *exposure, purchase, consumption,* and *termination* (e.g., Wansink, 2006). The first stage can result from *cue exposure*, such as the sight and smell of food when it is directly available, as well as internal factors, such as hunger sig-nals, which regulate food intake. The second stage, *purchase*, involves indi-vidual choice, which is influenced by reward aspects of food, as well as learning and memory process. This stage is also greatly impacted by the wide availability of unhealthy food, such as that found in fast-food outlets. The *consumption* phase includes evaluating the sensory aspects of the food, which form memories of its reward or aversion. The final stage is *termination*, which lasts as long as satiety signals prevail over competing external cues. This comprehensive perspective captures several pathways toward understanding individual eating behavior.

Food choice decisions are likely to be influenced by food prices, household incomes, the education and knowledge of decision-makers, tastes, and individual's energy requirements. However, the amount of food we eat is also influenced by environment. For example, consumption norms (what is an appropriate amount to eat) are influenced (biased) by reference points, such as package size, plate shape, and so on. The influences of these cues often occur outside of conscious awareness. Think of going to a restaurant. We tend to believe that a typical restaurant portion size represents the appropriate amount to eat, when in fact it may be much larger than appropriate. People are also biased by the "health halos" that accompany labels and tend to overeat when foods are labeled as "low fat," or perceived as healthier versus less healthy (e.g., Subway vs. McDonald's). Research suggests that we eat more with our eyes than our stomach. Overweight people use more external cues (plate is empty) than internal cues (no longer hungry) to stop eating (Schachter, 1971).

When faced with food, people respond differently than when faced with other purchases. The desire for health and indulgence represents a clash. Consumers wish to satisfy seemingly contradictory desires. For example, in the face of the pleasure that Cinnabon promises, consumers suspend more rational thought and are drawn to the indulgence of it. The promised pleasure distracts from thoughts of a food's fat or caloric content. These biases suggest that perhaps people do not need more nutrition information, but information about their own behavioral tendencies and how they may be more easily managed through decisions.[4]

Throughout this book, I will argue that increasing consumer well-being requires changing the personal environment. For example, serving food off the stove or counter (rather than at the table) reduces multiple servings a person consumes by 30% (Wansink, 2006). Being aware of errors/biases will not always help to avoid them, and relying on cognitive control and willpower is often disappointing. For some, it may be easier to change their environment than to change their minds. A personally controlled environment can help people more effortlessly manipulate their consumption and lose weight. Other examples include repackaging

---

[4]Most people know that an apple is better than a candy bar. Yet, people find maintaining a healthful pattern of behavior quite difficult.

food into single-serving containers, or storing tempting foods in less convenient locations, and so on. Throughout this book, I will offer such examples that can help individuals control their eating behaviors.

A NEED FOR A MULTIDISCIPLINARY APPROACH

The understanding of eating behavior and obesity can be likened to the Buddhist parable of the blind men and the elephant. One blind man feels the tusk, inferring that elephants are hard and sharp-edged, like a blade. Another touches the soft, flexible ear and concludes that elephants are quite elastic. A third imagines massive strength from grasping the pillar-like structure of the leg. The perspective of each person touching the elephant is valid, as far as it goes. But no one understands the whole beast. Our scientific understanding of obesity will be more accurate if we take a multidisciplinary perspective.

The challenge of studying obesity is highlighted in Figure 1.1, which shows the critical role of various systems in shaping individual decision making and lifestyle choices. As shown, obesity can be studied on different levels, from individual genetics to social environment, and each level is the traditional domain of a different discipline. This means that a better understanding of obesity may require interdisciplinary approaches.

FIGURE 1.1   Levels of Analysis of Obesity

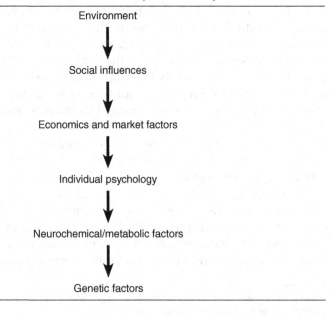

FIGURE 1.2   Economics and Psychology as Applications to Eating Behavior

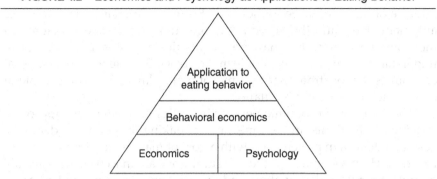

For example, a study of food prices provides an important explanation for the increase in obesity but does not explain why obesity appears to move through social networks. At the individual level, neurobiology may explain why some people prefer French fries to carrots. However, individual lifestyle choices are not completely independent of the social environment and norms. In short, the obesity epidemic results from a system with various parts that interact in a complex way that cannot be reduced to a single mechanism (Hammond, 2009).

This book attempts to use an interdisciplinary approach to better understand eating behavior and guide interventions to improve public health and overall well-being. It is designed to provide students with a foundation to explain why consumer food choices often conflict with their desire for good health and the barriers for making healthy diet choice by individuals. The discussions draw from several disciplines, including behavioral economics, nutrition, and public health, for understanding the relationships between a number of socioeconomic, nutritional, and behavioral factors on food intakes and health outcomes. Economics helps in understanding the role of food prices and household incomes on food consumption decisions. Psychology is interested in factors such as individuals' motivation to change lifestyle, belief about health, and degree of self-efficacy for encouraging healthful eating (see Figure 1.2).

A BRIEF INTRODUCTION TO BEHAVIORAL ECONOMICS

The book utilizes *behavioral economics* as the overarching conceptual framework to discuss the root causes of obesity. This relatively new field blends insights from psychology and economics. Behavioral economics is a generalization of *rational choice theory*, which incorporates concepts of rationality, willpower, and self-interest in a systemic way. The basic premise of behavioral economics is that humans are hard wired to make judgment errors and they need a "nudge" to make decisions that are in their own best interest. Behavioral economics provides a framework to understand when and how people make errors. Basic tenets of behavioral economics demonstrate that the environment plays an important role in eating and body weight regulation.

The traditional economic perspective relies on a "market" approach, in which individuals are assumed to be making autonomous decisions based on their own preferences, with a goal of maximizing individual satisfaction. However, many of these assumptions are inaccurate and simply do not fit what we know about individual behavior from public health. Human beings have limited cognitive abilities and limited willpower. Conscious and unconscious factors influence people's decisions in ways that cause us to act against our own best interest. As will be discussed in later chapters, biases, gut feelings, and habits often compete with deliberate consideration of information. Although individuals may be aware of the factors contributing to obesity, their everyday lifestyle choices do not reflect this knowledge. Rather, these choices are often made in an unconscious and a more impulsive manner. Because of this, individuals frequently make decisions that depart systematically from the predictions of economists' standard rational model. Behavioral economics attempts to understand these departures and, more generally, integrate psychologists' understanding of human behavior into economic analysis. Identifying ways in which behavior systematically deviates from optimality can then generate new insights into the underlying choice mechanism.

Behavioral economics suggests that we cannot always rely on revealed preferences (what people actually choose) as a guide for personal well-being. Standard economics normally assumes that revealed preferences are identical to preferences that represent the person's true interests. For example, when you choose chocolate over vanilla ice cream, you reveal a genuine preference for one flavor over another. However, there are many situations in which the choices people make do not reveal a true preference. For instance, several factors, such as passive choice, environmental cues, marketing, and present bias, tend to increase the gap between revealed and normative preferences. For example, people who eat popcorn at the theater tend to consume more than what they say they will eat, thus indicating a disconnect between revealed and normative preferences. The simultaneous prevalence of obesity versus the tremendous amount of money spent on diets and health clubs also reveals this disconnect. In situations like these, revealed preferences cannot be a reliable guide to normative preferences. The following chapters will describe factors that explain why our actual preferences deviate from our true preferences.

The body of literature discussed in this book illustrates the fact that satisfaction will not always be best achieved by allowing consumers to choose what they want, when they want it. Sometimes, people may be made better off by being given a restricted choice set, or by having their choices "guided" in the right direction. For example, many feel that the policy to ban smoking in public places is a good idea and has helped many people to quit smoking. In the context of food, consider the popularity of small snack packages, which help consumers control the amount of food they consume. Policies that eliminate problematic cues or promote counter-cues are potentially beneficial because they combat compulsive use while imposing a minimal inconvenience and restrictions on deliberate rational users. Moreover, self-control problems lead to *internality* ("harm to self"), which occurs when a person underestimates or ignores a consequence of his or her own behavior for himself or herself. Internality is one of the key rationales for public policy intervention in the context of addiction.

USING BEHAVIORAL ECONOMICS TO REDUCE OBESITY

As noted earlier, we often behave in ways that are inconsistent with our own stated desires. In the case of weight loss, we may tend to engage in overeating and fail to live up to some self-imposed ideal of eating behaviors. While individuals suffer from decision biases and self-control problems, they also have the capacity for self-regulation in a flexible and goal-directed manner through deliberate and effortful acts of willpower. This text will illustrate the usefulness of behavioral economics as a solution to problems that predictably arise from individual behavior. The discussion shows that many of the same decision errors that produce self-destructive behaviors can actually be used to improve an individual's health.

Self-control problems refer to an internal struggle dealing with choice over time. For example, Thaler and Shefrin (1981) formulate self-control problems as pitting the long-term preferences of a "planner" (or long-term self) against the short-term desires of a "doer" (or short-term self). This can also be framed as conflict between immediate gratification versus long-range consideration. Thus, self-control problems may arise when strong desires temporarily block the long-term self's ability to exert control over the short-term self. This formulation challenges the picture of the unified self as an optimizing single person. This means that there exists a gap between declared intentions and actual behaviors, where people seem to act against their best judgment. Successful use of self-control strategies allow individuals to choose differently than they would based on immediate preferences. In such cases, restricting an individual's choice is often a useful strategy to avoid temptation (e.g., placing alarm clock on the other side of the room so the person has no choice but to get up and turn it off and thus avoid oversleeping). In the context of eating behavior, Wansink (2006) demonstrates that when a jar of candy was placed within reach, participants consumed significantly more than the control group where the jar was placed 6 feet away.

POLICY IMPLICATIONS

There are two ways of thinking about influencing behavior. The first is based on the standard rational model. That is, influencing what people consciously think about by increasing knowledge and awareness (known as the *reflective system*). This approach assumes that the individual is a rational agent who surveys the situation to see what the various options are and then does a quick cost-benefit analysis of those options in order to choose. The second approach is to alter the context within which people act (known as the *automatic system*). This type of intervention is similar to the "nudge" outlined by Thaler and Sustein (2008), which often involves small changes to the choice environment. For example, one intervention tried to encourage school children to make healthier choices without alienating students by reducing their perceived choices. In a school cafeteria, what kids choose depends on the order in which the items are displayed (Thaler & Sustein, 2008).

From a policy perspective, the issue is how to motivate people to perform and maintain behaviors that are in their own best interests but that can be bothersome or difficult to do, such as eating properly, exercising, and moderating bad habits. The policy goal is to transform the environment in which food choices are made into one that supports healthy lifestyles. By focusing on creating conditions that help individual choices and behavior, we come to an argument in favor of some paternalism. The main justification for paternalism is that people have self-control problems. People want to behave differently from the way they are inclined, and they are willing to pay for it.

Some health policy analysts claim that the twenty-first century will be the century of behavior change. An understanding of the forces that shape individual health behavior choices is an essential ingredient in the development of effective policy to promote obesity prevention. Focusing on key behavioral economic factors that explain eating behavior, this book offers perspectives on how these psychological and economic factors may influence maintaining healthy habits over the long run. Any policy aimed at changing how people eat has to account for how these decision variables might change and how people will respond to that change by altering their lifestyles.

CONCLUSION

Rational food decisions often involve trade-off between short-term gains of sensory pleasure and longer term gains of health and wellness. Findings from behavioral economics research suggest that even when people are motivated to make healthy choices, external constraints in the decision-making process can prevent them from choosing optimally. Most of us prefer immediately gratifying short-term pleasure over our long-term goal of eating healthy. The following chapters will discuss several reasons why people go astray when making food decisions. Errors in choices arise from systemic decision biases, emotion, and the limits of cognitive capacity.

2

Explaining Eating Behavior

INTRODUCTION

Obesity is ultimately the result of an imbalance between energy consumption and energy expenditure. People gain weight if they eat too much and exercise too little.[1] However, data overwhelmingly suggest that the pattern of population weight gain over the past generation has been due largely to an overconsumption of energy rather than a decrease in physical activity patterns. This chapter describes an integrated approach toward eating behaviors and obesity. The approach is similar to an integrated biopsychosocial model. The fundamental assumption is that eating behaviors are consequences of the interplay of biological, psychological, and social factors. Food intake is regulated by a complex interplay of physiological, environmental, and cognitive factors. Changes in these factors might be responsible for increased food intakes and obesity. The focus will be on those factors that influence eating behavior outside of homeostatic need, which is an important avenue to address obesity prevention and control.

THE OBESITY EPIDEMIC

Obesity is arguably the most serious public-health problem facing the United States. Obesity has increased dramatically in the past few decades to such an extent that the Centers for Disease Control and Prevention (CDC) now refer to excess weight and obesity as an "epidemic."[2] Overall, about two-thirds of the U.S. population is estimated to be overweight or obese. In 2007–2008, 68.0% of U.S. adults were overweight, of whom 33.8% were obese (Flegal, Carroll, Ogden, & Curtin, 2010). This is in unfortunate contrast to the goal set a decade ago that no more than 15% of

---

[1]The basic formula for gaining and losing weight is well known: a pound of fat equals 3,500 calories.
[2]The word epidemic means that there is a higher-than-usual prevalence of a condition, and also it suggests that the condition is spreading rapidly.

people would be obese in 2010 (Healthy People, 2010). More Americans are obese than smoke, use illegal drugs, or suffer from ailments unrelated to obesity.[3]

Obesity is globally estimated to be the seventh leading cause of mortality (Ezzati et al., 2002). According to the United Nations, more people, or roughly the same number, are overweight than undernourished. About 1 billion people in the world are overweight and more than 400 million are obese, compared with 850 million who are underweight. The dual burden of malnutrition and overweight currently observed in many developing countries reflects a transition stage of the obesity epidemic.

WHAT IS OBESITY?

Obesity is weight that endangers health because of its high body fat relative to lean body mass. Obesity is not actually about weight gain, it is about excess gain in fat. In fact, the medical and health concerns over the rise in humans' average weight revolve around the extra weight being predominantly fat, and fat is intimately tied to energy. Positive energy balance leads to an increase in energy stores, which generally translates into an increase in adipose tissue.

A good screener for obesity is the Body Mass Index (BMI).[4] Obesity is diagnosed when BMI passes a defined threshold: People are said to be *overweight* if their BMI is greater than 25 and *obese* if their BMI exceeds 30. BMI is considered to be a good indicator of obesity for the general population (Table 2.1). It is a widely accepted index that correlates with percent of body fat. A substantial body of evidence shows that BMI is positively associated with both morbidity and mortality.[5] Both very low BMI (extreme thinness) and high BMI are associated with greater morbidity and mortality.

---

[3]See http://www.cdc.gov/obesity/data/trends.html

[4]In 1998, the federal government adopted the World Health Organization's definition of adult obesity: a body mass index (BMI). BMI is a person's weight in kilograms, divided by height in meters (or BMI = [Weight in Pounds] ÷ [Height in inches]^2 × 703). For example, a 20-year-old woman, 5 ft 6 in and weighing 132 lb (BMI = 132 ÷ [66]^2 × 703 = 21.3) is within the normal weight range. A BMI calculator can be found at http://www.nhlbisupport.com/bmi. A person is defined as anorexic with a BMI cutoff of the fifteenth percentile for the person's age and gender in addition to indicators of negative body image (the individual considered herself to be overweight or was trying to lose weight).

[5]Studies show a U- or J-shaped relationship between BMI and mortality, with individuals at very low and very high weights at increased risk.

TABLE 2.1 Classification of Adults According
to Body Mass Index

Category	Value
Underweight	<18.5
Normal range	18.50–24.99
Overweight	25.00–29.99
Obesity	⩾30.00
Mild (Class I)	30–34.99
Moderate (Class II)	35–39.99
Severe (Class III)	⩾40.00

There are obvious drawbacks to using the BMI, the most important being its inability to distinguish fat from bone and muscle mass, so it can misclassify some people. BMI may overestimate body fat in athletes and others who have a muscular build. Similarly, BMI may underestimate body fat in older persons and others who have lost muscle mass. In the elderly, a low BMI probably reflects low lean body mass. Aging is associated with a loss of lean body mass and an increase in abdominal adiposity. Thus, a healthy BMI may be misleading if the individual has low muscle mass and thus a greater proportion of fat. Another limitation of the BMI is that it cannot describe where the fat is located around the body. There is increasing recognition that certain patterns of body fat distribution contributes to obesity-related disease risk independent of overall adiposity.[6] For instance, carrying excess abdominal fat increases one's risk of ill health and mortality even with BMI held constant. Abdominal body fat as indicated by waist circumference is an independent predictor of type 2 diabetes.[7] Therefore, it is important to monitor measures of both overall and regional adiposity, such as body weight and waist circumference (Hu, 2008).

---

[6]For example, if you are in the 25–29.9 BMI range but your waist is less than 35 inches (for women) and 40 inches (for men), your odds of developing type 2 diabetes and other chronic weight-related illnesses are significantly lower than people with the same BMI but bigger waistlines. The same applies to those with BMIs ranging from 30 to 34.9. For those with BMIs above 35, waistline is less important in the risk calculation. Evidence shows that in men over 65, waist-to-hip ratio is a stronger predictor of coronary heart disease (CHD). Most likely, people with low BMI and a large waist have more visceral adiposity, whereas those with a high BMI but relatively small waist have more lean body mass. Thus, a larger waist circumference appears to be a better measure of adiposity in older people.

[7]Of course, insulin resistance is influenced by many factors, including age, diet, physical activity, body weight, and genetic variations. Increasing physical activity along with appropriate dietary change is the most effective way to increase an individual's insulin sensitivity.

THE PHYSIOLOGY OF WEIGHT CHANGE

Living organisms can be viewed as biological systems that cycle energy through themselves. *Metabolism* is the means by which they cycle energy to perform the necessary functions of life. Metabolism refers to the entire range of biochemical processes that transform nutrients into internal energy. Energy is released by the oxidation of ingested food. The total energy expenditure per unit of time is called the *metabolic rate*.[8] Total energy expenditure consists of three components: (1) *resting or basal metabolic rate*, (2) food digestion, and (3) muscular physical activity. The sum of all these components equals total energy expenditure. A change in any one of these components may result in a change in total energy expenditure.

Resting metabolic rate (RMR) is the number of calories that your body normally burns while resting. The RMR reflects the cost of maintaining body functions, including temperature, at rest. It is the minimum amount of energy needed for your body to function. In sedentary adults, the RMR accounts for 60% to 75% of total energy expended. RMR declines with age from the second to the seventh decade at a rate of 1% to 2% per decade. That is why we gain weight as we age. (Between the ages of 20 and 50 years, the typical adult in westernized countries such as the United States gains ~25 lb in weight.[9])

Food digestion[10] accounts for 10% of total energy expenditure, mainly due to the energy costs of nutrient absorption, processing, and storage.

Finally, physical activity typically accounts for 15% to 30% of the total energy expenditure. Physical activity is the most variable element and contributes significantly to interpersonal differences in weight.

Different people have different metabolic rates, and there are many reasons for these individual differences. One is that muscle supports a higher metabolic rate than fat. Therefore, two people can weigh the same, but the one with a higher percentage of body muscle will have a higher metabolic rate. Metabolic rate is also affected by the amount eaten. If

---

[8]The major categories of food components that usually are accounted for when determining the caloric value of food are fat, carbohydrate, and protein. The vast majorities of our calories come from fat, carbohydrate, and protein. A calorie requirement calculator can be found at http://www-users.med.cornell.edu/~spon/picu/calc/beecalc.htm

[9]The aging process is associated with a decrease in muscle mass, and muscles are metabolically more active than fat. Our muscles can be considered as being the energy powerhouse of our body, where most of our calories are burned. Our muscles shrink as we age. If we keep our caloric intake exactly the same as we get older, those unburned calories end up as fat. Evidence suggests that exercise helps the muscle cells get bigger and stronger.

[10]For example, a *stick* of *celery* has negative calories because eating and digesting celery use more energy than its calorie content.

someone reduces food intake to lose weight, that person's metabolic rate would decrease. Metabolic rate can also be increased by exercise.[11]

GENETIC CAUSES OF OBESITY

An important question in obesity research is why is there a recent, rapid increase of obesity in the United States. Because this increase has occurred over a relatively short time period, genetic factors are not seen as playing a predominant role in the current obesity epidemic. The human gene pool is unlikely to have changed dramatically within a few decades. Instead, overweight and obesity are the result of an interaction of genetic, metabolic, lifestyle, diet, environmental, and psychological factors. The level and impact of these factors can vary from individual to individual, and these individual differences are affected by genetic factors.

Individuals differ in their susceptibility to becoming overweight. Most notably, obesity is more prevalent (10 times more likely) in persons whose parents, brothers, or sisters are obese (Schousboe et al., 2004). Studies in identical twins have clearly demonstrated that genetics play a major role. For example, nonidentical twins raised together were less similar in weight than identical twins raised apart (Schousboe et al., 2004).

The nature and nurture interactions associated with obesity are thought to occur after conception but before birth. The womb is the baby's first environment. Maternal nutritional imbalance and metabolic disturbances during pregnancy could affect gene expression and contribute to the development of obesity and diabetes mellitus of offspring in later life (Packard, 2009). Nutritional exposures may result in lifelong remodeling of gene expression (these are known as *epigenetic changes*). The genes inherited from parents may be turned on and off and the strength of their effects change by environmental conditions in early development (Packard, 2009). So, events very early in life can set young children on an obesity trajectory that is hard to alter by the time they are in kindergarten. Research studies among Pima Indians showed that siblings born after the mother developed type 2 diabetes had a higher BMI throughout childhood and were almost four times as likely to develop diabetes as siblings born before the diagnosis (Dabelea et al., 1998). The intrauterine environment of a woman with diabetes overnourishes the fetus and may reset the offspring's satiety set point, and make the individual predisposed to eat more.

---

[11]It should be noted that generally obese people do not suffer from a very low metabolic rate. Obese people have higher metabolic rates than normal-weight populations (Garrow, 1988).

Individuals who as fetuses suffered food deprivation[12] are more likely to accumulate fat and to gain weight, as well as to suffer from type 2 diabetes and cardiovascular disease (Hu, 2008).

In sum, genetic factors may determine who in a given population is more susceptible to a damaging environment. It is likely that gene-environment interaction(s), in which genetically susceptible individuals respond to an environment with increased availability of palatable energy-dense foods and reduced opportunities for energy expenditure, contribute to the current high prevalence of obesity. With obesity, we are in a classic situation of genes loading the gun and environment pulling the trigger (Bray, 1998).

EVOLUTIONARY EXPLANATIONS FOR OBESITY

Evolutionary reasons have provided a framework for understanding eating and overeating. Two central evolutionary tenets are the *mismatch paradigm* and the concept of *homeostasis*.[13] Both theories propose a genetic susceptibility to weight gain, although each provides a different rationale. In either case, we can identify the general environmental contexts that promote overeating.

The mismatch paradigm states that our adaptive[14] responses lead to overeating and an accumulation of excess adipose tissue (Power & Schulkin, 2009). Our biology, which was shaped by millions of years of evolution, is not prepared for our modern society, which has profoundly changed how we eat. The ability to store surplus energy as fat has now become one of the biggest health risks for many human populations.

Humans, like most animals, have evolved to eat more than necessary to meet their immediate nutritional needs and provide a buffer against future periods of food scarcity (Pinel, Assan, & Lehman, 2000). Our bodies evolved to discount delayed food and to eat as much as

---

[12]This is known as biological programming, which refers to marginally incomplete fetal development, of which low birthweight is a nonspecific marker. Malnutrition retards brain development and interferes with the development of vital organs like the gut, heart, and lungs, making them weaker and more prone to later failure. Some of the damage is reversible if proper nutrition is restored. Fogel argues that malnourished humans wear out more quickly and are less efficient at every age.

[13]These tendencies also have been described as the "thrifty genotype" hypothesis (Neel, 1962), which suggests that humans tend to conserve energy and to eat in excess when they can. Genes controlling human behavior have been selected for environments characterized by frequent periods of food scarcity. The "thrifty genotype" hypothesis suggests that there is a mismatch between biology and modern life because famines are rare in developed countries, but our genes favor fat deposition.

possible, conserving the energy consumed within the body as much as possible. Those who could eat a lot and build up reserves of fat had an advantage when lean times came. So they survived and transmitted this ability to their descendants. Whereas this regulation system was once adaptive in an environment characterized by scarce food supplies, it has become maladaptive in the modern environment characterized by an abundance of food. The human eating system did not evolve to cope with the continuous exposure to highly tempting foods, such as French fries, hamburgers, or chocolate cookies.[15]

The maladaptive response of overeating under conditions of abundance is often explained in terms of difficulties to resist the temptation of the immediately rewarding value of palatable foods. Indeed, given modern temptations, it is impressive how many people remain in normal weight range. Thus, from the biological perspectives, weight gain and obesity are the inevitable outcome of the mismatch between our evolutionary endowment and modern lifestyles in developed countries. The greater the mismatch between the "expected" environment and the actual one, the more likely our adaptive responses will come up short.

The homeostatic model states that hormonal signals will regulate eating behavior and body weight. Our body has checks and balances that, for most of human history, allowed the body to match energy input to energy output. Our body uses hormones and neurotransmitters to ensure that the calories we consume match the calories we burn. For example, when one feels hungry, the body is out of homeostatic balance in terms of available energy. When your stomach has been empty several hours, a chemical called *ghrelin* (the "hunger hormone") is released into the bloodstream. Ghrelin levels rise just before mealtime and fall after we eat. Ghrelin is made in the stomach and tells our brain when it's time to eat. As levels of ghrelin rise, the chemical reaches a part of the brain called the *hypothalamus* (a regulator of appetite), where ghrelin initiates a chain reaction that we experience as hunger. We look for food and start eating.

How does the body know when to stop eating? Our stomach stimulates the release of another chemical, *cholecystokinin*, or CCK, which also acts on the hypothalamus. CCK fosters a sensation of fullness, or satiety.[16] Evidence shows that fasting ghrelin levels are lower in obese individuals and fail to decline after a meal, and this may contribute to their overeating (Dagher, 2009).

———————

[14]In evolution, adaptation refers to a characteristic that addressed a challenge that the organism's ancestor faced. If the challenge no longer exists, or has changed, then the selected characteristic may no longer be adaptive.
[15]Like animals in captivity, human beings in the modern environment confront novel circumstances daily. Many have no adverse effect, and indeed are beneficial.

Our body maintains a long-term reserve of energy, mainly in the form of fat, to draw on between meals or when food is scarce. When a person misses a meal, the body begins metabolizing, or breaking down, stored fat into components called fatty acids, which can be burned as fuel. The body has ways of detecting the optimal level of fat stores. This optimal level is determined by genetics and metabolism, as well as environment. *Leptin*, a hormone that is secreted by fat cells, makes the hypothalamus more sensitive to satiety signals from the gut. When fat stores are high, more leptin is secreted, thus we are inclined to eat less. A very small number of people who are obese do not produce enough leptin.[17] If you are not making enough leptin, you may still feel hungry, even though you are putting on weight. Insulin modifies food intake by inhibiting eating and by increasing leptin release, which also can inhibit food intake.

Moreover, our physiology tends to set the brain in one of two modes: *homeostatic stable state*, which helps us maintain a steady weight, and *reward-seeking state*, which encourages us to seek food. For instance, after significant weight loss, leptin levels drop. When there is a deficiency of leptin, the areas of the brain associated with reward-seeking become more active. Researchers (Rosenbaum, Sy, Pavlovich, Leibel, & Hirsch, 2008) have shown that leptin mediates changes in areas of the brain that regulate the emotional and cognitive aspects of eating after weight loss. In a study, the researchers recruited overweight volunteers who agreed to a calorie-restricted diet aimed at shedding 10% of body weight. Using fMRI scans, the researchers looked at how the volunteers' brain reactions to seeing food changed after weight loss. They found that there was more blood flow to

---

[16]Eating fast could interfere with the signaling system that tells your brain to stop eating because your stomach is swelling up. Eating fast may provide insufficient time for the full effect of satiety signals to operate as food reaches the intestine. Fast eating is a behavior that might have been learned in infancy and could be reversed, although this might not be easy. Thus, one way of increasing satiety is by slowing down the consumption of food and concentrating on the perception of every bite, which is typically fast in the obese individuals (Otsuka et al., 2006). The evidence shows that trying to slow down mealtimes for children would have an impact on future obesity rates. So, the old wives' tale about chewing everything 20 times might be true.

[17]In 1994, Rockefeller University researcher Jeffrey Friedman and his colleagues published a landmark paper in *Nature* that identified a hormone called leptin (Greek for "thin") produced by the obese (ob) gene. Friedman showed that mice lacking the ob gene do not produce leptin and become extremely obese. After both normal and ob-deficient mice were injected with synthetic leptin, they became more active and lost weight. High levels of leptin activate nerve cells in the brain and create a feeling of fullness, while low levels signal hunger. Friedman also showed that humans who lack the ob gene and eat large amounts do not experience that feeling of fullness and end up extremely obese.

areas of the brain known to be involved in the emotional control of food intake. After weight loss, the participants had an increase in the emotional response to food and a decrease in the activity of brain systems involved in restraint. However, when they restored leptin to these volunteers by giving them injections of the hormone, the brain response changed. The study concludes that even though leptin is not an anti-obesity hormone, drugs that would stimulate leptin signaling could potentially facilitate the maintenance of weight loss.

An alternative explanation is that bodyweight is regulated to a "set-point." The set point is a sort of thermostat that sets an optimal weight for each person. When it has plenty of food to burn, it turns up the "furnace" and burns out fat reserves faster. When it has less food to burn, it turns down the furnace and burns it more slowly and efficiently. If you eat too little, the body goes into conservation modes and makes it even tougher to burn off the pounds. This efficiency helped our ancestors survive famines and barren winters.

The set-point theory predicts that (1) weight gain can occur effortlessly, and the accumulation of adipose tissue proceeds with little physiological resistance, and (2) weight loss occurs with difficulty, and the loss of adipose (fat) tissue is resisted tenaciously. In other words, human body defends against long-term energy deficits much more vigorously than it does against long-term energy excess. The classic semi-starvation study conducted by Keys et al. (1950) provides some support for a set-point theory in humans. After losing 25% of their original body weight over a 6-month period, male volunteers experienced powerful urges to eat.

The set-point theory suggests that it is difficult for the obese to lose and then maintain weight loss. If bodyweight is defended, efforts to achieve and maintain weight loss may be thwarted by a strong, biological drive to return to a higher set point. However, Berridge (2004) points out that there is a mismatch between the set-point prediction and the observed reality. Instead of having set points, we have "settling points" for body weight. Even individuals of normal and stable body weight often employ deliberate efforts (diet and exercise) to maintain their weight.

In addition, modern foods are radically different from those of our ancestors (plant foods and high fiber foods). Foods are processed and easier to eat; they break down more quickly in the mouth. Processing means removing the elements in whole food—like fiber and gristle—that are harder to chew and swallow. The result is food that does not require much effort to eat. Because this kind of food disappears down our throats so quickly after the first bite, it readily overrides the body's signals that should tell us, "I am full."

Many modern foods also are generally high in sugar and fat, and they tend to be low in fiber (thus easily digestible) and high glycemic. We show considerable preference for sweet foods[18] and overindulge in eating them, especially when they are cheap. For example, we can indulge in preferred foods to an extent far greater than our physiology was ever likely to have been exposed to in the past. High glycemic foods[19] favor fat deposition. By definition, eating these foods results in a rapid increase in the absorption of glucose into cells, where it is oxidized in cellular metabolism or converted into an energy-stored molecule (glycogen or fat), which causes adipose tissue to accumulate. High glycemic foods also encourage "grazing," or eating between meals, because they produce less satiation and thus a lower reduction in appetite. Restricting diets to low glycemic index foods has been shown to be successful at promoting weight loss if total food is not restricted.

In summary, a significant contributor to the increase in human obesity is due to a mismatch between the adaptive biological characteristics of our species and the modern environment, which has changed dramatically from the one under which we evolved. Food is plentiful, and it does not require extreme or prolonged exertion to obtain. Furthermore, the food industry plays upon our physiological responses to food in order to motivate us not only to choose certain foods but also to eat larger amounts of those foods. We are paying the price for our success at modifying our environment in ways that increase our access to food, especially high-calorie food, and at the same time reduce our necessary energy output. In this stimulus-intense modern environment, the need to control one's impulse has become increasingly important.

------

[18]Humans naturally like sweet things, because sugar is a good source of calories, and we dislike bitter things, because bitterness is a cue to toxicity.

[19]Satiety may be increased with the intake of low glycemic index (GI) foods (the slow-release carbohydrates). For example, chickpeas have GI of 39 versus the instant mashed potatoes with GI of 122. Evidence suggests that low GI foods (55 and under) are beneficial for weight control and reducing the risk type 2 diabetes. Low GI foods have the ability to promote satiety and delay hunger, and reduce fluctuation in blood sugar levels. Epidemiological studies have shown that a low GI dietary pattern is associated with lower triglycerides and higher HDL cholesterol levels. Dieticians recommend that whenever possible replace highly processed grains, cereals, and sugars with minimally processed whole grain products. However, a GI fails to tell us the amount of digestible carbohydrate. For example, watermelon has a very high GI. But a slice of watermelon has only a small amount of carbohydrate per serving. A related way to classify foods that takes into account both the amount of carb in the food and its impact on blood sugar levels is known as the glycemic load (GL). A food's GL is determined by multiplying its GI by the amount of carbohydrate it contains. In general, a glycemic load of 20 or more is high and 10 or under is low. For more information, see this site: www.glycemicindex.com.

THE DEVELOPMENT OF FOOD PREFERENCES

Food choice is influenced by the taste of food, and a greater liking of foods, in general, is a cause of overeating. Our acquired likes and dislikes guide our food choices and the amount of food we consume. Research shows that these acquired flavor likes can act as a risk factor for overeating and obesity (Yeomans, Tepper, Rietzschel, & Prescott, 2007). For example, a strong preference for sweetness ("sweet tooth") is usually accompanied by subjective experience of a need for sweet foods in the daily life. Moreover, obese individuals with a preference for dietary fat have been demonstrated to be less prone to retrain their diet. Thus, the way we acquire flavor[20] preferences and individual differences in the ability to acquire such preferences may be a risk factor for development of obesity. The following describes several mechanisms through which flavor preferences develop.

We have innate tendency to like sweet tastes and dislike bitter tastes. For infants and children, the general rule seems to be the sweeter the better. For example, sweet medications are more likely to be accepted by children. This preference for sweet tastes has been explained in a number of ways: the reliable relationship in nature between a sweet taste and safe food (e.g., ripe fruit); the fact that many nutritious foods are rich in sugar; and acceptance of sweet-tasting mother's milk at birth.

Similarly, bitter-taste aversion has been explained as an innate avoidance of items that have the potential to be poisonous, since most poisons have bitter tastes. However, these initial aversive responses can be reversed if ingestion of bitter-tasting foods fail to lead to illness, or leads to a positive experience (e.g., the effects of alcohol or caffeine).

Social learning also facilitates flavor preference development. Social learning refers to modified eating behavior due to the mere presence[21] of others. For instance, studies show that people eat more when in groups than alone. Social factors play an important role in our initial exposure to foods, which helps us to learn what is safe. For example, social learning explains the acquisition of a liking for spicy food by children in certain cultures who are exposed to spicy foods in meals that are consumed by adults. The social environments in which children grow up enable them to develop a sense of how foods should taste.

----

[20]Flavor is not the same as the primary taste system. Taste receptors on the tongue are tuned to detect five taste qualities: salty, sour, bitter, sweet, and umami (having a rich taste). Similar to primary colors, these basic tastes are mixed to form complex tastes, or flavor. From an evolutionary perspective, these taste qualities likely evolved to solve a basic nutritional problem, such as detecting beneficial foods and rejecting harmful ones. Unlike primary senses, flavor involves complex integration of multiple sensory inputs relating to the experience of food or drink in the mouth.

The knowledge of food preference development has important implications for changing children's dietary habits. Infants' innate food preference and their development of taste perception provide an obstacle to the acceptance of certain types of food.[22] We cannot easily change the innate preference for sweets and avoidance of bitterness, which makes it difficult for children to eat nutritious foods when these foods do not taste good to them. Presentation of a novel item of any kind may initiate a fear response. "Picky/fussy" eaters consume inadequate variety of foods, which leads to nutrient deficiency.

Successful and continuous positive experiences with a food item will lower the child's reluctance to eat it. It is suggested that up to 15 positive experiences may be required for successful acceptance of a food into a child's habitual diet (Yeomans et al., 2007). The more the people around the child consume the novel food, the more willing the child will be to try it. Young children learn to accept food through observing significant others. Expression of this fear also tends to decrease with age.

Finally, children's flavor preferences are strongly influenced by the mother's dietary choice when she is pregnant and nursing. The flavor-learning occurs during prenatal experiences from the mother's diet through the amniotic fluid. This flavor-learning continues when infants are breast-fed, since human milk is composed of flavors that directly reflect the foods, spices, and beverages ingested by the mother. For example, infants whose mothers consumed more fruits and vegetables during pregnancy and lactation were more accepting of these foods (Mennella, Jagnow, & Beauchamp, 2001). Thus, the child's flavor preference is partly shaped prior to the first taste of solid foods.

EATING FOR HUNGER VERSUS EATING FOR PLEASURE

Why do people tend to overeat in spite of somewhat obvious future health implications? Why, under some circumstances, do we eat more? As noted above, we must eat to survive. However, in modern times, among well-nourished populations, most food consumption occurs for reasons other than acute energy deprivation. It is widely acknowledged

---

[21]Similarly, the mere exposure effect argues that repeated exposure leads to increased liking through familiarity. Early life exposure of more "ethnic" foods will increase acceptance of these foods.

[22]An important factor explaining this innate preference is known as food neophobia that helps children avoid eating potentially poisonous foods. Food neophobia is an element of "picky/fussy" eating. Whereas "picky/fussy" eating is the rejection of a large proportion of familiar foods, food neophobia is defined as the rejection of foods that are novel or unknown to the child.

that an important stimulus for eating is not hunger, but the anticipated pleasure of eating determined by the sensory qualities of palatable food. Lowe and Butryn (2007) suggest that the presence of food may stimulate psychological hunger just as the absence of food causes physiological hunger. There has been a significant increase of the sensory stimulation produced by the taste, smell, texture, and appearance of food, as well as its availability. On the other hand, the satiety signals produced by the physiological hunger have remained essentially unchanged. The effect on the appetitive system is a net average increase in the reward value and palatability of food, which overrides the satiety signals, and the tendency to be over stimulated by food, and overeating. Thus, human eating behavior is regulated not only by homeostatic mechanisms but also by the food reward system. Understanding this reward system may help us understand the factors that influence the excessive food intake associated with obesity.

Figure 2.1 shows that the appetitive system for food consumption can be regulated by physiological hunger and *hedonic*[23] *hunger*. The homeostatic system responds to energy signals and hedonic hunger responds to food cues (e.g., the sight and smell of food) in the absence of an energy deficit. Research indicates that these two systems interact to provide signals with food intakes (Dagher, 2009).

For instance, appetite-stimulating hormones, such as ghrelin and insulin, act directly on the dopamine system, which encourages us to seek food. The dopamine system substantially influences our food consumption. Thus, our physiological system motivates us to search for food. When you crave a bowl of chocolate ice cream after dinner, in the absence of physical hunger, it is your dopamine reward system that gets excited. In many situations, this desire to eat can override the need to eat, leading people to overeat and contributing to obesity.

An important aspect of the appetitive system (Figure 2.1) is that individual differences in sensitivity to food reward account for food intake. The individual differences may lead some people to be more responsive to particular classes of foods, which leads to a lifetime pattern of food choices and eventual weight gain. These sensory factors include food palatability, sensory-specific satiety, stress, and mindless eating (discussed below). These factors explain why homeostatic regulatory systems are superseded in the "*obesogenic*" environment, and they are important in obesity prevention. The key to effective obesity prevention

---

[23]The term hedonic derives from the Greek term for "sweet," relating to pleasure. Hedonic experiences have been linked to the classic motivational theory that people approach pleasure and avoid pain.

FIGURE 2.1   Motivations to Eat

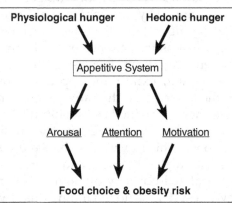

is to understand how the sensory factors can be controlled by cognition (self-control) so as not to override satiety signals.

The following sections describe several causes that motivate food consumption (aside from the need for energy). The discussion shows that it does not require pathology to overindulge in food. Modern foods are easy to obtain and the availability of palatable foods increases hedonic hunger that can lead to overindulgence. The later chapters show that slight differences in reward system reactivity explain why some people overeat, whereas others do not.

Food Palatability

Eating is an important source of pleasure. People's intake varies as a function of *palatability*. Palatable food (tasty food) refers to those foods that have the capacity to stimulate the appetite and prompt us to eat more. They tend to be sugary, fatty, and salty. Palatable food may motivate eating in excess of what is necessary for homeostasis. The better-tasting the food, the more we will eat. Thus, palatability is a key factor in promoting overeating and obesity.

Palatable foods, especially those high in sugar and fat, can activate the reward circuits in the brain and tends to stimulate eating. The prime suspect here is the *opioid system*. Blocking the opioid system reduces the pleasure derived from tasty foods, and thus calorie consumption. This suggests that the malfunctioning of the opioid system may contribute to the development of eating disorders. For example, individuals suffering from reward-deficiency syndrome show a lack of pleasure from consuming a regular amount of food; they need to eat an excessive amount of attractive foods to perceive eating as a rewarding activity

(Volkow & Wise, 2005). Chapter 8 will discuss the parallel between the overconsumption of desired foods and drug addiction.

Sensory-Specific Satiety (Food Variety)

Sensory specific satiety is defined as a decrease in appetite, or the subjective liking for the food that is consumed, with little change in the hedonics of uneaten food (Roll, 2005). As a result of sensory-specific satiety, when people consume a variety of foods,[24] they tend to overeat. A greater variety of food leads people to eat more than they would otherwise. So, being full and feeling sated are separate matters.[25] The recovery of appetite or the motivation to eat is apparent to anyone who has consumed a large meal and is quite full, and does not require additional energy or nutrients to meet their daily needs, but decides to consume additional calories after seeing the dessert cart. Small changes in the sensory properties of foods are sufficient to increase food intake. For example, subjects who were presented with different shapes of pasta showed increased hedonic ratings and increased energy consumption relative to subjects eating only a single shape of pasta (Rolls, 1986). Similarly, in an experiment where people were offered different varieties of sandwiches in sequence, they consumed 15% more calories than those who were repeatedly offered the same one (Rolls, Roe, Halverson, & Meengs, 2007).

The operation of long-term sensory-specific satiety may also increase malnutrition. It involves a decrease in palatability for foods consumed repeatedly. For example, U.S. soldiers given a supply of prepared food rations in a limited variety lost more than 10 pounds in a matter of a month because they reduced their caloric intake so drastically (Rolls, Rolls, Rowe, & Sweeney, 1981).

This weight loss actually necessitated adding a greater variety of foods to the prepackaged meals to increase intake. Such lack of variety (monotony) suppresses eating through the mechanism of sensory-specific satiety, the rapid development of satiation when one's food supply is monotonous (Polivy, Herman, & Coelho, 2008).

If variety increases intake of less healthy foods, it may also increase intake of healthier foods. Children provided a variety of healthier or less healthy foods increased energy intake for both healthy and less healthy

---

[24]It is important to note that choosing a variety of nutrients-dense foods helps to ensure adequate intakes nutrients that are needed for healthy living.

[25]The propensity to seek out and respond to food variety may be an evolutionarily advantageous phenomenon that may have arisen to ensure a balanced nutrient intake (Epstein et al., 2009). Food variety has consistently been shown in animals and humans to increase energy intake.

foods. Thus, it may be possible to take advantage of food variety to improve healthy eating by increasing access to a variety of healthy foods while simultaneously reducing access to a variety of less healthy alternatives.

Habituation

Habituation is another concept that can help understand the influence of sensory influences (rather than energy depletion) on eating. The terms habituation and sensory specific satiety are often used interchangeably. Habituation is a basic form of psychological adaptation that occurs in the nervous system. Habituation is a decrease in response to a stimulus after repeated presentations. For example, a novel sound in your environment (such as a new ring tone on your phone) may initially draw your attention or even become distracting. After you become accustomed to the sound, you pay less attention to it and your response to the sound will diminish.[26] This diminished response is habituation. Individual differences in habituation provide a framework to understanding factors that regulate food intake behavior, and preventing or treating obesity (Epstein et al., 2009).

The presentation of a novel food may disrupt the process of habituation and slow down the rate of habituation. This is likely what happens when one consumes a variety of food during a meal. Varied foods act as novel stimuli.[27] If you taste a food, it is stored briefly in short-term memory, and if a second taste of that food matches the information in short-term memory, then a reduction in stimulus processing will occur. Because short-term memory has a limited capacity, attending to a new food stimulus would remove the information about the habituating stimulus from short-term memory. This would slow or prevent habituation.

The same mechanism occurs if a nonfood environmental stimulus causes disruption of attention, and thus occupies short-term memory, while someone is eating. For instance, shifting attention from food to the

---

[26]Habituation is an important reason for "not crying wolf" when nonthreatening animals come close. By habituating to less important signals, an animal can focus its attention on the most important features of its environment. A good example of this is species that rely on alarm calls to convey information about predators. In this case, animals stop giving alarm calls when they become familiar with other species in their environment that turn out not to be predators.

[27]A simple food item could be an apple or a glass of milk, while a combination food could be a pizza or a soup or stew, which involves combining several foods into a final food product. Modern food industry produces multisensory effects. Foods rich in combinations of sugar and fat are more common now than ever. These foods give us more sensory stimuli and lead to excessive consumption.

environmental stimulus would slow habituation. Many people purchase large buckets of popcorn to eat during a movie, larger amounts than they would be likely to consume if they were just eating popcorn without watching a movie. The movie stimulus serves to remove information about food stored in short-term memory, thus slowing down the rate of habituation.

Habituation could be a risk factor for the development of obesity. A slower rate of habituation should predict greater energy intake. For example, obese children and adults show slower rates of habituation than their leaner peers. Research also shows that obese adults and children have an explicit memory bias for food stimuli when compared with non-obese peers, as assessed by free recall tests (Epstein et al., 2009). Memory is critical to the regulation of eating. Without memory of eating, there is a reduced inhibition to eat. Rozin et al. (1998) showed that amnesic patients would consume multiple meals within 10–30 minutes of a previous meal because they did not remember they had eaten. Overweight people consume a greater variety of foods than lean people, and overweight people who enter weight control programs are more successful if they reduce the variety of high energy density foods they consume.[28] Watching television is another behavior that has been related to obesity, and this leads to the obvious recommendation to limit distracting stimuli during eating, such as watching television or reading the newspaper, given that distracting stimuli disrupt the habituation process and lead to increased energy intake.

Stress

Human eating behavior is similarly sensitive to the effects of stress, with the specific outcome depending on the nature of the stressor (acute or chronic) and individual differences. Stress promotes eating of palatable foods (sweet comfort foods) in about 30% of the population (Dallman, 2010). Psychological (e.g., interpersonal, ego-threatening, and work-related) stressors have been linked with an increase in food intake and snacking. These aversive aspects of stress are suggested to increase desire for the hedonic soothing effects of eating palatable foods.

Stress may drive the consumption of highly caloric comfort foods.[29] Moreover, through repeated experiences, individuals may learn that

---

[28]Similarly, in addiction literature it is known that the self-administration of two drugs in combination may increase the desired effect of one drug or both drugs (e.g., the combination of cocaine and heroin known colloquially as a "speedball.")

[29]Evidence has shown that sweet preference is associated with personality trait (e.g., lack of assertiveness). Lack of assertiveness implies a lower self-confidence and lower self-esteem. Thus, sweet taste and comfort foods act as compensation for lower life satisfaction.

eating these foods can reduce some of the unpleasant effects of stress and thus, with further stressor encounters, individuals may "self-medicate" through eating "comfort foods." Evidence shows that elevation of stress level increases the likelihood of energy-food consumption (Dallman, Pecoraro, & la Fleur, 2005). Van Strien, Herman, and Verheijden, (2009) suggest that perhaps we should try to explain the current obesity epidemic from an emotion perspective. Consuming comfort foods may stimulate pleasure centers in the brain, thus regulating stress-induced systematic arousal. Stress-induced amygdala activation can be dampened by the ingestion of energy-dense food. In a world where people often feel under stress, food is an escape. Specifically, intake of palatable or preferred food leads to the release of dopamine and endogenous opioid peptides within the central nervous system. Purchasing indulgent food is an inexpensive form of entertainment.

Technological changes have brought about a progressive shift away from physically demanding tasks to knowledge-based work requiring an enhanced mental effort. The increased cognitive demand is associated with emotional stress (such as a burnout), which is known to favor overconsumption of comfort food as a coping mechanism. As individuals turn to comfort foods to alleviate stress, the continued failure to cope with stressors may promote the development of obesity.

Stress might also increase the likelihood of experiencing depressive symptoms. Depression has been associated with increased comfort food consumption.[30] Depression is also associated with reductions in physical activity (Ströhle, 2009). Depressed individuals are rather self-neglecting and lead less healthy lifestyles, including poor diet and lower physical activity. Gender also appears to be an important moderator of the association between depression and obesity, such that there is a positive association of increased BMI with and depression among women (McCarty et al., 2009).

However, stress induced from the threat of physical harm or discomfort (illness or fear of injury) decreases food intake. Emotional overeating is an inappropriate response to distress. Distress is associated with physiological reactions designed to prepare the individual for a fight-or-flight reaction. Stress inhibits gastric motility and promotes the release of sugar into the bloodstream, thereby suppressing feelings of hunger. Thus, it has

---

[30]Previous studies have shown that depression can lead to eating disorder. However, the causal relationship between obesity and depression is murky and is possibly bi-directional. For example, depressed individuals often take antidepressant medication, which enhances appetites and thus overeating. Also, leptin resistance may contribute to depression, in which leptin resistance causes altered appetites and overeating (Beydoun & Wang, 2010).

been postulated that the "unnatural" response of emotional overeating is a learned behavior (Wardle, 2007). It occurs in people who cannot distinguish hunger from other aversive internal states, possibly as a result of inappropriate learning experiences early in life.

It is shown that that physical activity is associated with the release of so-called "feel-good" endorphins. Thus, adding physical activity into one's daily life could serve to promote the same "reward" as high-calorie foods, but without the detrimental health consequences in the long term. Also, evidence shows that those with a good mood tend to desire to consume healthier, low calorie foods (Wardle, 2007).

Food Cues

Exposure to attractive food cues increases food consumption in animals and humans, even when they are already satiated. In fact, the presence of food cues (a meal presented to be eaten) can be more potent than signals of satiety. The presence of food cues stimulates a desire for a particular food, as well as increasing intake.[31] For example, Fedoroff, Polivy J, and Herman (1997) found that the smell of cookies baking increased cookie craving and cookie consumption for all participants (though more so for chronically dieting restrained eaters).

Another trait shared by many people who are either overweight or obese is their tendency to keep eating beyond the point of hunger. In the 1970s, Stanley Schachter, a Columbia University social psychologist, became convinced that overweight people did not respond appropriately to internal signals, such as hunger, satiety, or a need for fuel. He hypothesized that overweight people ate in response to external cues, rather an internal signals. His theory came to be known as *"externality."* The sight of food was exerting more pull on the overweight population than any internal messages reporting an absence of hunger. The externality theory recognized the power of cues. These cues amplify the rewarding aspects of highly palatable food. People differ in how they respond to external stimuli; some are more impulsive, while others are better at avoidance behavior.

MINDLESS EATING

Many of us eat whatever is put in front of us. *Mindless eating* refers to behaviors that occur without awareness, are initiated without intention, tend to continue without control, and operate with little effort. Eating turns out to be one of the most mindless activities we do. It is a behavior over which the environment has more control than do individuals. Moreover, people are often unaware of the amount of food they have eaten or of the environmental influences on their eating. For example, a recent survey showed that adults underestimate what they eat by 800 calories (Wansink, 2006). These incorrect estimations usually are done unconsciously.[32]

The concept of mindless eating behavior is supported by studies that demonstrate the impact of the environmental context and food presentation on eating. The amount of food eaten is strongly influenced by factors such as portion size, food visibility and salience, and the ease of obtaining food. When people are served a portion of food, they tend to assume that the portion size defines the reasonable meal amount to eat.[33] Increasing portion size by 50% resulted in higher daily energy intakes that were sustained for an 11-day period (Rolls et al., 2007). Reducing portion size leads to overall reductions in energy intake.

In studies of children's behavior, Barbara Rolls has found that very young children are far less affected by portion size than older children. When 3-year-old preschoolers were given lunches with a small, medium, or larger portion of macaroni and cheese, portion size did not influence consumption: the kids ate a certain quantity and then stopped, regardless of how much food was on the plate. By contrast, Rolls found that with 5-year-olds, greater portion size led to greater intake. Such findings suggests that as children grow older, they become less responsive to internal hunger and satiety cues and more reactive to environmental stimuli.

In a series of clever experiments, Wansink (2006) showed that eating is often done with little awareness. For example, Wansink cleverly manipulated bowls of soup to refill themselves, hidden from the participants. Those eating from the self-refilling bowls ate 73% more soup than did those eating from normal bowls of the same size, but believed that they had eaten the same amount and felt no more sated than those eating from normal bowls. Similarly, Wansink (2006) found that presenting popcorn in large packages versus medium-sized containers led to 45.3% more consumption, and even when the popcorn was stale and bad-tasting, large portions produced 33.6% more eating than did medium-sized portions.[34]

Rozin, Kabnick, Pete, Fischler, and Shields (2003) documented that the French paradox is partly explained by the fact that the French eat less than Americans. French portion sizes are smaller in comparable restaurants, for example, a McDonald's grilled chicken sandwich weighs 175 grams

---

[31]The human response to environmental stimuli is known as priming. For example, North, Hargreaves, and McKendrick. (1997) showed that when they played French music in a wine store people bought more French wines, and when they played German music people bought more German wines, with little or no awareness of the effect of the music on their purchases.

in Philadelphia and 155 in Paris. Also, people in France, on average, spend more time eating a meal than do people in the United States; yet French people consume fewer calories per meal even though they spend more time eating. A study (Kahneman, Schkade, Fischler, Krueger, & Krilla, 2009) comparing wellbeing of 800 women in Columbus, Ohio, and 800 women in Rennes, France showed a striking difference in the BMI of these women. The average BMI in the Columbus group was 28; in the Rennes group, it was 23. One important explanation was the incidences of focal eating. Sixty percent of the French women surveyed reported that, when eating, it was the main activity in which they engaged. Only 30% of American women reported eating as a focal activity.

Characterizing eating as mindless (or automatic) behavior does not mean that human beings cannot bring eating under volitional control. People certainly can refuse dessert or resist the temptation of the chocolates in the jar on the desk. All automatic behaviors can be controlled temporarily. But the amount of effort required to refrain from eating when food is present is substantial, and it is nearly impossible to sustain over the long term. Chapter 11 will discuss the concept of self-control and mental effort involved in refusing tempting food. The idea of mindless eating suggests that to reduce consumption we should decrease the accessibility, visibility, or quantities of foods to which people are exposed and reduce the cues in our environment that encourage eating. These approaches include limiting access to ready-to-eat foods and limiting the availability of snack foods in schools and workplaces. The understanding of our eating as mindless behavior helps to avoid blaming our lack of willpower to maintain a diet and recognize our automatic eating in response to environmental cues.

In conclusion, obesity is the result of thousands of small choices that have the outcome that caloric intake exceeds the decision maker's caloric expenditure. Wansink's work (2006) demonstrates that environmental cues influence the frequency and quantity of what people eat and that people do not typically recognize these cues. This body of work shows that making consumption decisions more mindful can change people's eating behavior. More importantly, the view of eating as a mindless

---

[32]Informally known as the eye-mouth gap syndrome—the underestimation of the amount of food you eat and the overestimation of the types of food that you consume.

[33]According to the US Department of Health and Human Services, many foods today contain double or more calories compared with how they were routinely served 20 years ago.

[34]The size of plates, bowls, and glasses in our homes has also steadily increased over the years, and the serving size of some entrees has virtually doubled in recipe books. Hint: if you would like to lose weight, get smaller plates, buy little packages of what you like, and don't keep tempting food in the refrigerator.

behavior suggests that to avoid overeating we should focus on shaping the food environment (e.g., serving potato chips in small, single portions rather than a large bowl). It reinforces the common sense notion that if you're not paying attention to what you're eating, you're likely to eat more than you realize.

CONCLUSION

Obesity reflects an imbalance between energy intake and expenditure that is mediated by the interaction of energy homeostasis and hedonic food intake behavior. The increase in body weight is mostly due to the fact that people are simply eating more calories of food, rather than because they are exercising less. This chapter described several reasons, including genetic, physiological, dietary, and psychological factors. Modern temptations to eat and keep on eating are stronger than in the past because the modern foods are highly palatable (they contain high levels of sugar, fat, and salt). They are also easy to obtain. All of these factors may play into the brain reward systems in ways that let us succumb to the desire to eat more.

The chapter also described two motives for eating. We eat to prevent true energy deprivation, which is referred to as homeostatic hunger. The second motive for eating is driven by the reward value of palatable foods in the absence of energy need. The reward value of food may either override internal signals of satiety or lead to the development of a separate motivation to consume palatable foods (so-called hedonic hunger). The concept of hedonic hunger increases our understanding of poor weight control in that hedonic processes overcome homeostatic regulation. Moreover, certain individuals are vulnerable to succumb to weight gain. Their unique biological and behavioral features, as well as their responsiveness to the environment, encourage weight gain. The remainder of this book will discuss these risk factors from a behavioral economic perspective.

3

Some Basic Economic Concepts

INTRODUCTION

This chapter provides some basic microeconomic concepts and tools as they apply to resource allocation decisions, including the market mechanism, efficiency, and optimization. The main objective is to enhance students' understanding of economic behavior and demonstrate the role of economics in decision making. The chapter also explains what behavioral economics is and how it is different from standard economics. In later chapters, the economic principles discussed here will be applied to behavioral issues, such as overeating and obesity.

WHAT MOTIVATES PEOPLE?

The fundamental human motive is the desire to obtain pleasure and avoid pain. People and animals are motivated to avoid pain and attain pleasure, and they organize their actions around those twin pursuits. That is, people evaluate each alternative by balancing imagined pleasure against imagined pain and select the alternative that promises greater average pleasure. It should be noted that pleasure does not necessarily imply hedonism. It comes from many sources, including acts of virtue or relief from pain. Likewise, pain arises from a sense of injustice, or frustration from falling short of a goal. There is also pleasure in relief from pain and suffering (e.g., relief from hunger or thirst).

Economics assumes that people make decisions based on their own self-interest, preferring wherever possible to maximize their total satisfaction. The pursuit of self-interest is a fundamental economic motive. In the words of Adam Smith, "It is not from the benevolence of the butcher, the brewer, or the baker that we expect our dinner, but from their regard to their own interest." (Smith, *Wealth of Nations* 1776/1977, Bk I, chap 2, p. 14). The idea is not that people act selfishly and without altruism, but rather that in the pursuit of self-satisfaction, individuals produce goods and services of value to others, providing mutual gain from their exchange.

THE CONCEPTS OF PREFERENCE AND UTILITY

Preference,[1] a concept in economics and psychology, is subjective desirability. It is essential to the decision-making process. Preference prepares our actions. Preference means imagining the future. That is why different people who are presented with the same options make different choices. People who think about behavior in terms of preferences tend to assume that understanding a person means understanding that person's preference.

Economists model people's preferences using the concept of *utility*. Utility is generally synonymous with satisfaction. It measures the extent of goal achievement. Utility is not the same as "pleasure." The concept of utility respects the variety of human goals. It represents whatever people want to achieve. Some people do not want "pleasure" as much as they want other things (such as virtue, productive work, respect, or love—even when these are painful things to have). Each person's conception of utility or well-being can admit selfish, altruistic, spiteful, or even self-destructive behavior. For example, smoking yields personal benefits to the smoker, such as "comfort," a "friend" in times of stress, and participation in a mutually enjoyable activity with one's peers.

An early introduction of the utility notion into the social sciences was suggested by the English philosopher Jeremy Bentham (1748–1832). Bentham viewed utility as the net sum of positive over negative emotions. For him, utility referred to pleasure and pain, the "sovereign masters" that "point out what we ought to do, as well as determine what we shall do." (Kahneman, 2000). For Bentham, utility was commensurate with happiness (experienced utility, or enjoyment), which was measured as an individual's inner happiness—directly and cardinally measurable, like length or temperature (Kahneman, 2003).

Later on, the neoclassical economists—such as William Stanley Jevon (1835–1882)—extended Bentham's utility concepts to explain consumer behavior. Jevon thought economic theory was a "calculus of pleasure and pain," and he developed the theory that rational people would base their consumption decisions on the extra marginal utility (MU) of each good. In short, many *utilitarians* of the nineteenth century believed that utility was a psychological reality—directly and cardinally measurable, like length or temperature.

Since feelings were meant to predict behavior but could only be assessed from behavior, economists realized that utility cannot be

---

[1]Taste is a form of preference. In economics, preferences are inferred from choices and assumed to reflect utilities. In psychology, preferences are thought to be constructed in order to make a choice. For example, Thaler and Sunstein (2008) show that the design of decision environments nudges people to construct their preferences.

measured in an objective fashion. For them, the mind was inaccessible—the brain was just a black box. Thus, neoclassical economists sought to explain behavior in more psychologically neutral terms. This process culminated in the development of *ordinal utility* and the theory of *revealed preference perspective* (also known as *decision utility*), according to which utility represents as an index of preference rather than of happiness. More precisely, utility refers to how consumers rank different goods and services. Under this approach, consumers need to determine only their preference ranking of bundles of commodities. For example, one could rank pictures in an exhibition by order of beauty without having a quantitative measure of beauty. Revealed preference theory (or decision utility) simply equates unobserved preferences with observed choices. Thus, utility is inferred from observed preferences. Moreover, these thinkers postulated that humans are rational. When we make decisions, we are supposed to consciously analyze the alternatives and carefully weigh the pros and cons.

LIMITATIONS OF THE RATIONAL CHOICE MODEL

In economics, the rational model is a starting point. Rational choice in economics means that individuals understand their own preferences, make perfectly consistent choices over time, and try to maximize their own well-being. People are rational agents who set goals and pursue them intelligently by using the information and resources at their disposal. The agent surveys the situation to see what the various options are. Then she or he does a quick cost-benefit analysis of those options, in order to pick the best one. Rational choice implies choosing according to long-term outcomes rather than short-term ones.[2] Many economists believe that useful insights into our behavior can be gained by assuming that we act *as if* governed by the rules of rational decision making.

Humans can be brilliant, but they can also be stupid (such as by getting hooked on life-destroying drugs). For instance, many humans are very committed to worthy long-term goals, such as eating healthy food and saving for retirement, and yet, in the moment, when faced with temptations, we cave in and forego our long-term plans. This demonstrates

---

[2]Rational choice does not have to be sensible or adaptive. It only has to result from a weighing up of the costs and benefits as the decision-maker sees them. So it is rational, if often unwise, for a person to choose short-term gain over the avoidance of a possible long-term pain. A young person with a short time-horizon may simply not care about life after 30. In the midst of an alcohol binge, an individual may not even care about the prospect of a hangover the following day. These are unwise choices but they are not irrational.

the separation of preference from action. Such inconsistency in human behavior presents a challenge to the principle of rational choice, according to which consumers would be able to attribute proper value to delayed rewards when it enhances the chance of maximizing their long-term gain (i.e., forgoing an unhealthy food now in the interests of better health later).

To be truly rational, we would need, at a minimum, to face each decision with clear eyes, uncontaminated by the passion of the moment, with appropriately dispassionate views of the relevant costs and benefits. A rational agent would be able to exert self-control and deny immediate rewards in the interest of delayed but bigger rewards (such as, for example, a slim body, improved physical health, and increased longevity).[3]

However, the weight of evidence from psychology and neuroscience suggest otherwise. We can be rational on a good day, but most of the time, we are not.[4] The economic rational model is built on an inaccurate view of human nature. Furthermore, Elster (1999) notes that the pursuit of interest can hardly be called rational if it is based on irrational beliefs, such as wishful thinking and self-deception.[5] So, for a choice to be rational, it should be well-grounded in the evidence available to the agent. For example, a person whose preferences are very present-oriented, in the sense that he does not take much account of future consequences of present behavior, would not rationally invest many resources in finding out what those consequences might be.

BEHAVIORAL ECONOMICS

Behavioral economics, which blends insights of psychology and economics, is rapidly becoming part of the microeconomics mainstream. It is about understanding the roots of decision-making biases in the brain. Behavioral economists have shown the limits of the classical economic

---

[3]One might say that the drug addicts are not rational. In fact, studies show that taking drugs will induce a deficit of rationality by impairing individual ability to defer gratification, that is, from being unable to take account of future consequences of personal behavior. The person with a short time-horizon is trapped.

[4]Alan Greenspan noted in his Congressional testimony in 2008, that he was shocked that markets did not work as anticipated. "I made a mistake in presuming that the self-interests of organizations, specifically banks and others, were such as that they were best capable of protecting their own shareholders and their equity in the firms."

[5]Wishful thinking—when people would like a certain proposition to be true, they end up believing it to be true.

model, which assumes that individuals are efficient, rational, utility-maximizing creatures.

Herbert Simon (1955) was an early critic of modeling economic agents as having unlimited information processing capabilities. He proposed that decision makers should be viewed as *bounded rational*,[6] and offered a model in which utility maximization was replaced by *satisficing* (a decision-making strategy that defines what is an acceptable or adequate outcome). He suggested the term "bounded rationality" to describe a more realistic conception of human problem-solving capabilities. In 1970s, cognitive psychologists[7] began to map bounded rationality, by exploring the systematic biases in judgment and economic decision making. They took maximization of utilities and logical rules of probability judgment as benchmarks and used conformity or deviation from these benchmarks as a source of systematic biases (Kahneman, 2003). Behavioral economics is a generalization of rational choice theory, which incorporates limits on rationality, willpower, and self-interest in a systemic way. The rational model can play the important normative role of guiding people toward better decisions, ones that accord more fully with their real objectives.[8]

Neuroeconomics

While behavioral economics provides a rich conceptual model for understanding individual choice, neurobiologists provide tools for the study of our decision-making mechanism. The new field of *Neuroeconomics*[9] examines the neural bases of decision making (McCabe, 2003). It explores such phenomena as how the brain tends to release pleasure-inducing

---

[6]Bounded rationality implies biases in acquiring information, biases in processing information, biases in transmitting information, and biases in receiving and storing feedback.

[7]Cognitive psychology—finding errors of perception or logic. This field studies how people think and reason in terms of processes that, although not "observable," could at least be described.

[8]Economist Stigler once said that to take root, an economic theory must meet the triple criteria of generality, manageability, and congruence with reality. In his view, ideas compete with one another in the intellectual marketplace, and the most general, manageable, and realistic must inevitably triumph. In this view, behavioral economics provides fruitful insights and new ways to describe and even shape behaviors.

[9]In 1996, this term was invented by McCabe in creating the name for a course on neurology and economics. One could also apply the term to a method in which the brain allocates its own scarce resources, and that in some sense is what is this study of the economics of the brain and the effect this has on behavior.

chemicals when it anticipates rewards and how emotions influence thinking. The insights from this field provide a conceptual framework to understand decision making.

Neuroscience, the study of the brain and nervous system, provides direct measurement of thoughts and feelings, and the neural basis of decision making. Neuroimaging technology allows researchers to detect changes in metabolism or blood flow in the brain while the subject is engaged in cognitive tasks. The aim of this approach is to validate mechanisms that psychologists uncover and to offer new interpretations of existing mechanisms. In general, the science of human behavior and how the brain creates this behavior is known as *cognitive neuroscience* (Gazzaniga, 2008).

The Brain as a "Black Box"

The traditional economic approach to study decision making is similar to the behavioral approach used by psychologists. The decision process has been for economists a "black box." The foundations of utility theory were constructed assuming that details about the functioning of the brain's black box would not be known. The person is seen not as a repository of mental states, but as a whole organism interacting with other organisms and with objects in the world. The person's mental states may be interpreted in terms of these interactions.

Throughout much of the first half of the twentieth century, behaviorists believed that the subjective inner states of mind, such as perception, memories, and emotions, were not appropriate topics for psychology. Mental states came to be known pejoratively as the "ghost in the machine." Behaviorism called instead for an exclusive emphasis on observable behaviors—acts that can be objectively seen, recorded, and quantified (LeDoux, 1996). Feelings, thoughts, plans, desires, motivations, and values—the internal states and personal experiences that make us human—were considered inaccessible to experimental science and unnecessary for a science of behavior.

The neuroeconomic theory of individual choice replaces the concept of a utility-maximizing individual who has a single goal with a more detailed account of how components of the individual—brain regions, cognitive control, and neural circuits—interact and communicate to determine individual behavior. From this perspective, decision making can be understood as the resolution of the interaction and often competition between different specialized neural systems (Sanfey et al., 2006). The understanding of choice in terms of competing brain regions reveals important insights about human behavior.

ECONOMICS, SCARCITY, AND CHOICE

Choice and decision making is a fundamental aspect of life, and the choices people make determine in part the quality of their lives. Economics provides a conceptual framework to understand how people decide to allocate their limited resources (e.g., money and time) among available alternatives to maximize happiness (total utility). Economists study the decisions people face when their wants cannot all be met at once. (e.g., we like to be thin and eat healthy, but we also like a slice of cheesecake.) Economic choices have important consequences for individual well-being, such as health, wealth, material possessions, and other sources of happiness. In the context of eating behavior, economics provides a framework to understand factors influencing everyday choices, which lead to positive energy balance and obesity.

Economists study problems of *scarcity*. Every decision to use resources has an *opportunity cost*[10] in that those resources cannot be used to produce benefits elsewhere. In a world of scarcity, choosing one thing means giving up something else. The cost of the foregone alternative is the opportunity cost of the decision.[11] Time is the ultimate scarce resource, yet we act as if we have unlimited time. Poor or rich, we all have 24 hours a day, 7 days a week. Thus, each of us faces the choice of how to spend our time. Time is relatively scarce for people with higher income, partly because their time is more valuable. So, to have lots of time, rich people hire other people to do their house chores. On the other hand, a nonworking person may spend more time on household production.

Sunk costs are those costs that are beyond recovery at the moment a decision is made. Consider for example an annual membership in warehouse clubs, such as Sam's Club. Once you have joined, the natural inclination is to buy enough stuff so that you can "recoup" the price of membership. The result could be overspending, even on things we do not need (e.g., 5-pound barrels of pretzels or 48 packets of instant oatmeal). In this case, the sunk cost is the motivation factor.

Economists recommend that we always consider opportunity cost, but ignore the sunk costs, in decision making. However, consumers tend

---

[10]What is the opportunity cost of being obese? Tosini (2008), focusing on American White women born in 1960–1964, shows that women who are obese at age 30 are more likely never to have been married by 7 percentage points, they are less likely to be divorced (conditional on having been married) by 4 percentage points, their husbands have earnings that are lower by 27%, and they have a much harder time finding a husband they like.
[11]For example, if a typical stay-at-home mother in the United States were paid for her work as a housekeeper, cook, and psychologist among other roles, she would earn over $100,000 a year. The typical mother puts in a 90-hour work week, working 40 hours at base pay and 52 hours overtime.

to do the opposite. We have all experienced the pervasive pull of sunk costs or commitment in some form or another, such as investment of time or money in a doomed project or relationship. The deeper the hole we dig ourselves into, the more we continue to dig.

Desperation is the mother of invention. Out of desperation comes efficiency. Efficiency requires addressing two questions: (1) "What is the value of my available choice?" and (2) "How much does each choice cost?" To be efficient, a system must value its available options, and valuation means estimating two things: the cost and the long-term returns associated with each option. Those that accurately estimate the costs and the long-term benefits of each choice will be more efficient than those that do not, and in the long term, those are the winners. Efficiency means the best long-term returns from the least immediate investment. Just like the "buy low, sell high" tip. Economics guide us to choose the best for the least. Your time and energy are limited and so your choice consumes precious resources. Choice also means loss (opportunity cost). All outcomes, including doing nothing, are choices.

The single property that all efficient systems require is goals—meaning that one cares about something. Without goals, a system cannot be efficient for the simple reason that it has nothing against which to gauge its ongoing performance. For example, in developing a project, you are confronted by the following questions: What do you want the project to do? In other words, what do you value and what is the budget? How do we choose which goals to pursue? Some of our goals are instinctive drives that come with our genetic inheritance, while others are subgoals that we learn (by trial and error) to accomplish goals that we already hold. Higher goals and values are adopted from the parents, friends, or acquaintances to whom we become "attached," at least in our earliest formative years. Subgoals play special roles to help us learn ends instead of means.[12]

In economics, we say that an economy is producing efficiently when it cannot make anyone economically better off without making someone else worse off. *Pareto Optimality* is a situation in which no reorganization or trade could raise the utility or satisfaction of one individual without lowering the utility or satisfaction of another individual. Pareto's principle captures a theory about how to operate efficiently in daily life. The practical implication is reflected in *the 80/20 principle*, which states that one

---

[12]For example, a business student expresses that the reason she is majoring in business is to make a lot of money, and the reason she wants to make a lot of money is that she believes money brings freedom and happiness. However, she may later on discover that she is happier helping another person than shopping.

can in general accomplish most of what one wants—perhaps up to 80% of the target—with only a relatively modest amount of effort—perhaps only 20% of expected effort. The principle is the observation that most things in life are not distributed evenly. For example, 20% of the input creates 80% of the result, or 80% of your sales may come from just 20% of your products. The obvious implication is that a small proportion of your efforts provide most of the result. Thus, we can make better use of our time by investing our efforts in the 20% that will get us 80% of the results we want to achieve.

A distinction is usually made between analyzing the consequences of a change and making judgment concerning the desirability of particular changes or policies. The former kind of analysis is called *positive economics*, whereas the latter is referred to as *normative economics*.

DEMAND AND SUPPLY

The theory of *supply and demand* shows how consumers' preferences determine consumer demand for commodities, whereas business costs are the foundation of the supply of commodities. Demand and supply analyses are important economic models used for determining price and predicting equilibrium, such as predicting the effect of a change in demand for a service.

Demand

Demand reflects consumers' final preferences. Economists define demand as the desire to purchase a good or service backed up by the necessary purchasing power. In economics, demand does not mean "want" or "need." Individuals may have many needs but if they lack purchasing power, they cannot demand goods. A need is the essence of fixed thinking: the amount of some commodity to be consumed is viewed as being fixed and independent of prices. When backed up by cash, the most urgently felt needs get fulfilled through the demand curve.

Consumers purchase goods and services for the satisfaction (utility) that they yield. However, some goods purchased by consumers do not fall into this category. For example, consumers do not get satisfaction directly from the purchase of auto tires or gasoline, but they are necessary to run their cars. The demand for these goods is a *"derived demand."* Thus, the demand for these goods depends on the demand for the goods and services they help to produce. In the same way, medical care services do not augment utility directly. The demand for medical care is derived from the more fundamental demand for health itself, which produces utility. Regular visits to the dentist may be undertaken in order to produce healthier teeth and gums in the future. In that sense, the patient is investing in dental care now in order to produce healthier teeth in the future.

The law of downward-sloping demand: The most fundamental rule of economics is that a rise in price leads to less quantity demanded. For most goods, it is reasonable to assume that demand will vary inversely with the price of the good. The higher the price, the less will be demanded. This holds true for a restaurant meal, a real-estate deal, a college education, illegal drugs, or just about anything else you can think of. When the price of an item rises, you buy less of it (which is not to say, of course, that you want less of it). There are normally two independent reasons for the quantity demanded to fall when the price rises: *substitution* and *income effects.* Price increase essentially reduces income and consumers then substitute lower priced items. Note that the price on the vertical axis of the demand curve diagram (Figure 3.1) usually refers to the real price of the good, which means its price relative to the prices of all other goods and services at the same time.

The determinants of demand: $D_x = f(P_x, P_y,$ income, taste, market size). In general, the following factors determine the demand for any goods and services: the good's own price, average income, prices of related goods, tastes, and population size. Changes in these factors, except the good's own price, will shift the entire demand curve. The quantities

FIGURE 3.1 Demand Curve

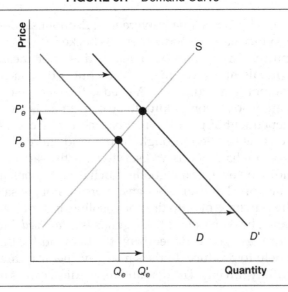

of goods and services that an individual is able to buy are constrained by the individual's available income. At any price, the quantity demanded will be greater than before, as income increases, with a resulting shift in demand curve. The demand for a good is affected by changes in the price of other goods. The demand curve will shift, but the direction and amount of the shift will depend on the nature of the good whose price has changed: the *substitute* or the *complement*.

Substitutes are goods with similar characteristics and which may be bought as alternatives to one another. For example, if product A and B are equally substitutable, then increase in the price of A will result in the demand for B to increase. It is suggested by some that alcohol and marijuana are economic substitutes. This means that if the price of one of these substances is raised, buyers will purchase more of the other. If so, increased barriers to alcohol use (such as enhanced law enforcement or higher prices) are likely to encourage some compensating increase in marijuana use.

Complements are goods that are generally used together so that increased consumption of one implies increased consumption of the other, such as cars and gasoline, or computers and software. If the price of one good rises, the demand for the other good will shift downward.

In general, demand shifts outward (it increases) because of an increase in income, rise in price of substitute, fall in price of complement, and increase in preferences for the good. Demand will shift inward (decrease) if these factors change in the opposite direction. As the population size and/or its structure changes, there will be corresponding shifts in the demand curves for many goods and services. A falling number of births will mean reduced demand for baby clothes and equipment; then demand for obstetric beds will fall. An increase in the elderly population will mean increased demand for residential home places, wheel chairs, and walking frames.

Market demand represents the sum total of all individual demands. The market demand is what is observable in the real world.

Supply

Business costs are the foundation of the supply of commodities. In general, the *supply curve* is determined by the good's own price, technology, input prices, and price of related goods. $S_x = f(P_x, P_y,$ technology, input prices) (see Figure 3.2). Again, changes in any of these factors, except the price, will shift the entire supply curve. If, other things being equal, the cost of producing a good increases, then at any given price its production becomes less profitable than before. Thus, we would expect the supply

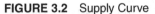

FIGURE 3.2 Supply Curve

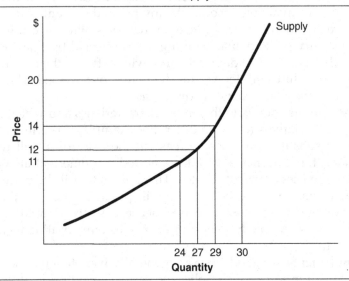

curve to shift to the left. Similarly, if a technological breakthrough or a fall in input prices means that the good can be produced at a lower unit cost, then at any particular price the production of the good is more profitable than before. In general, the supply curve will shift outward because of falling input prices and technology improvement. Supply will shift inward because of rising input prices.

Equilibrium

The *equilibrium*, or *market-clearing*, price and output are at the point where the demand and supply curves intersect. It is the price-quantity pair at which both buyers and sellers are satisfied. Equilibrium is a situation where there is no tendency for change (see Figure 3.3). At the equilibrium price of P_0, consumers are willing and able to purchase Q_0 units of, say, generic aspirin. Thus, both consumers and producers are perfectly satisfied with the exchange because both can purchase or sell their desired amounts at a price P_0. Such an outcome is desirable for two reasons: (1) individuals are making their own choices; (2) by not engaging in any more trades, individuals reveal themselves to be as satisfied with their economic lot as possible, given the resources with which they began.

Surplus or *excess supply* refers to the amount by which quantity supplied exceeds quantity demanded. *Excess demand* or *shortage* refers to the amount by which quantity demanded exceeds quantity supplied.

FIGURE 3.3 Equilibrium

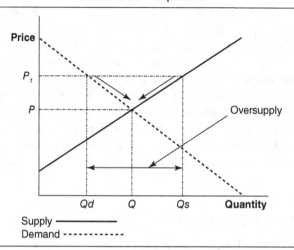

Supply ——————
Demand -----------

A *competitive equilibrium* is a situation where we have a set of market prices so that all markets clear, that is, there is no excess demand or excess supply. If the price was above P_0 in the figure, then the quantity demanded would fall short of the quantity supplied (i.e., excess supply), and market forces would cause the price to fall until the market clears. At the equilibrium point, the marginal benefit just equals the marginal cost, which implies that value is at its maximum and therefore the allocation is an efficient one.

The Concept of "Full Price"

To an economist, price is a broad concept. Price includes not only the monetary cost of purchasing a product but also the time and other costs associated with buying that product, as well as the health consequences and other costs from using the product. The full price of a good can be thought of as having four basic components: (1) monetary cost, (2) time cost, (3) potential legal cost, and (4) potential health cost. Overnight delivery, direct flight, and convenience stores all charge premiums because of the inherent value we place on our time. The 20 minutes you spend waiting for a table in a restaurant is part of the price, as are any nutritional consequences of the meal itself. The economist Kevin Murphy has calculated that a cheeseburger costs $7.95 more than a salad in long-term health implications (Murphy & Robert, 2005). While the restaurant's menu may list the price of the cheeseburger at $2.50, that is clearly just the beginning.

Time is money. Why do we often spend our money more wisely than our time? It is striking to note that how little thought we give to how we spend our time. Perhaps it's because we cannot save time; it passes whether we choose to spend it or not. You cannot bottle time and exchange it for an object or event. The value of time is higher during good economic times. Economic studies suggest that people tend not to take care of themselves in boom times (Miller, Page, Stevens, & Filipski, 2009). They tend to drink too much, eat fat-laden restaurant meals, exercise less, and skip medical check-ups because of work-related time commitments. So people work more and do less of the things that are good for them. Thus, people experience more stress due to the rigors of hard work during booms.

The Income-Consumption Curve

The analog to the individual demand curve in the income domain is the individual *Engle curve*. This curve plots the relationship between the quantity of a particular good or service consumed and income. As shown in Figure 3.4 below, holding preferences and relative prices constant, the Engle curve tells how much, say, health care a consumer will purchase at various levels of income. Note that the Engle curve is upward-sloping, implying that the more income a consumer has, the more health care he will buy each period. Most things we purchase have this property.

Why would someone buy less of a good following an increase in his income? A *normal good* is a good whose quantity demanded increases as income rises. An *inferior good* is a good whose quantity demanded falls as income rises. For example, if a consumer receives a large enough increase in income, then he may consume less Ramen noodles and switch to higher quality foods. Another way to distinguish between consumer goods is to classify them as *necessities* and *luxuries*. A good is defined as a luxury for a person if he spends a large proportion of his income on it when his income rises. A necessity, by contrast, is one for which he spends a smaller proportion of his income when his income rises. For example, Americans spend a smaller percentage of their expenses on food than any other country (7.2%) (Nord, 2009). By contrast, the figure was 22% in Poland and more than 40% in Egypt and Vietnam.

People with higher incomes spend more on health care. One of the key characteristics of all modern economies is that as they prosper, they collectively spend more money for health care (Feldstein, 2007). Like almost all commodities and services, health care seems to be a normal good, so that people's desire to use the good increase as their income increases. So the variation among countries per capita health care can be partly explained by the per capita income of a country.

FIGURE 3.4 The Engel Curve

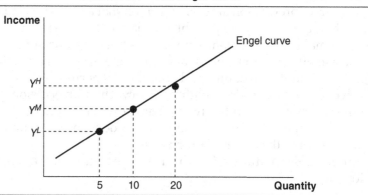

MARKET

A *market* consists of the buyers and sellers of a good or service. In economic theory, markets are fair (marked by impartiality and honesty)—free from self-interest, prejudice, or favoritism. Markets do not necessarily produce a fair distribution of income. A market economy may produce inequalities in income and consumption that are not acceptable to the public.

A market can be seen as a tool, or mechanism, for allocating resources in a society. Like any tool, a market can be used effectively to achieve certain objectives, but it is not effective in achieving others; similarly, it functions well in some contexts and poorly in others. A market is considered a desirable tool for allocating scarce resources for a number of reasons. The primary reason is that, under certain conditions, markets can lead to an efficient allocation of resources. That is, within a market system, if the conditions are met, goods are produced in a least-cost manner, the "optimal" mix of goods is produced, and those goods are distributed in a way that reflects the value individuals place on them.

Within a well-functioning market system, prices play a pivotal role in achieving the desirable outcome. Prices serve two important and distinct functions: on the supply side, prices ensure that resources are used in their most productive way (i.e., taking account of the opportunity cost, or what the resources could produce if used in another way), and on the demand side, prices ensure that goods go to those who value them most, in the sense that they are willing to pay for them (and pay more than other individuals).

The ideal competitive market consists of large numbers of profit-maximizing firms and utility-maximizing consumers. Under certain assumptions, the self-motivated behaviors of these economic actors lead to patterns of production and consumption that are efficient in the special sense that it would not be possible to change the patterns in such a way so as to make some person better-off without making some other person worse-off. Of course, efficiency is not the only social value. Human dignity, distributional equity, and economic opportunities are values that deserve consideration along with efficiency. Thus, on occasion, public decision makers may wish to give up some economic efficiency to protect human life, make the final distribution of goods more equitable, or promote fairness in the distribution process.

In general, conditions for an ideal competitive market include the following:

- A large number of buyers and sellers, no one of whom is so big as to have a significant influence on the market price.
- No collusion among buyers or sellers to fix prices or quantities.
- Relatively free and easy entry into the market by new buyers or sellers.
- No governmentally imposed restrictions on prices or quantities.
- Reasonably good information about prices and quality known to buyers and sellers.

A perfect competitive economy is efficient. The efficient market produces the bundles of outputs desired by consumers using the most efficient techniques and the minimum amount of inputs. Adam Smith (1976/1977) defined a decentralized free-enterprise economy as one in which each economic agent, consumer, or producer, act solely out of individual self-interest, seeking selfishly to maximize his or her own welfare.

MARGINAL UTILITY

Consumers gain satisfaction or utility from the goods they consume. As mentioned before, utility (psychological satisfaction) is a term that economists use to quantify benefits or losses as the person concerned sees them. In the context of choice, the utility of a particular option reflects the desirability of its consequences. For example, $100 will have different utility for a student than for a millionaire. Utility provides a single dimension on which to compare things that are very different—which is of course necessary when making a decision. We convert the various desirable attributes of each to a single scale so that they can be weighed against each other. That scale is utility. Thus, a *utility function* is a mapping between objective and subjective value. *Marginal utility* is a change in utility associated with a unit change in a good.

The *law of diminishing marginal utility* states that as the amount of a good consumed increases, the MU of that good tends to diminish. In general, the benefits derived from consuming the first unit of a commodity are high; subsequent units of that same commodity provide smaller benefits. Although total utility or benefits increase with additional units of the same commodity, the MU or benefit of additional units decline. The saying that you cannot have too much of a good thing means that for any good that you enjoy (say, a chocolate bar), higher consumption will always lead to greater utility, but not greater MU.

The rationale for the downward slope of demand is based on the principle of diminishing MU: each additional unit of the good is valued slightly less by each consumer than the preceding unit. If the consumer's extra utility declines with each extra unit purchased, then the consumer will only buy more if the price falls. Thus, the demand curve can be thought of as the marginal private benefit curve for an individual. The height of the demand curve shows the marginal value/benefit. For example, if the consumer already has purchased and eaten one hamburger, another unit may provide some extra satisfaction. However, a third unit will probably add less satisfaction than the second. This is an example of diminishing MU (see Figures 3.5–3.7).

Consumers are assumed to experience diminishing marginal utility as they increase consumption of any one good.

The Principle of Optimal Consumption Decision

The economist's rule of *"equality at the margin"* states that the MU of the last dollar spent on each good is exactly the same as the MU of the last dollar spent on any other good.

FIGURE 3.5   Diminishing Marginal Utility

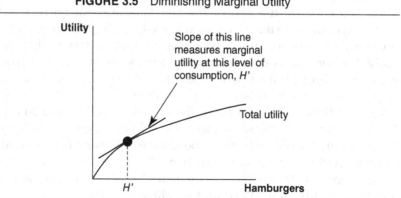

FIGURE 3.6   Total Utility Curve

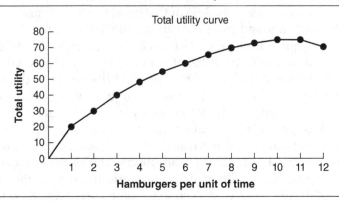

FIGURE 3.7   Marginal Utility Curve

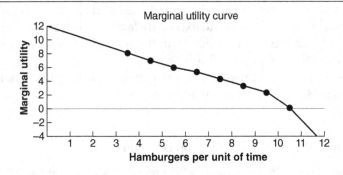

Note that MU becomes zero at the peak of the total utility curve.

What is the best way to allocate your leisure time? The principles of consumer choice suggest that you will make the best use of your time when you equalize the MU of the last minute spent on each activity. Suppose you want to maximize your knowledge in your courses, but you have only a limited amount of time available. You may find that an equal study time for each course will not yield the same amount of knowledge in the last minute. If the last minute produces a greater marginal knowledge in economics than history, you would raise your total knowledge by shifting additional minutes from history to economics, and so on, until the last minute yield the same incremental knowledge in each subject.

To use an example related to food, the relationship between MU and additional units of chocolate is shown in Table 3.1. To maximize total utility, the consumer will purchase 3 units if the price of each unit is $5, assuming the MU of the third unit is valued in dollars.

TABLE 3.1   Marginal Utility of Chocolate Bars

Chocolate Bars Eaten	Marginal Chocolate Utility	Total Chocolate Utility
0	0	0
1	70	70
2	10	80
3	5	85
4	3	88

ELASTICITY

A central analytical concept in demand theory is the *price elasticity of demand*, a measure of the responsiveness of purchase decisions to small changes in price. Price elasticity of demand equals the percentage change in the quantity of a good demanded that results from a 1% change in its price. A price elasticity of demand of 3 (absolute value) implies that a 1% increase in the price would reduce overall consumption by 3%.

$$\text{Elasticity}(E_D) = \frac{\%\ \text{Change in Quantity Demanded}}{\%\ \text{Change in Price}}$$

When a 1% change in price calls forth more than a 1% change in quantity demanded, the good has *price-elastic demand*. When a 1% change in price produces less than a 1% change in quantity demanded, the good has *price-inelastic demand*. In general, If $E_D < 1$, demand is inelastic, if $E_D > 1$, demand is elastic, and if $E_D = 1$, the demand is referred to as *unitary elastic*.

In general, three factors determine the size of price elasticity of demand: the availability of substitutes; the importance of the good in proportion to the consumer's budget; and whether or not the good is a normal good. Goods with ready substitutes tend to have more elastic demand than those that have no substitutes (e.g., a vaccine). For necessities such as food, fuel, shoes, and prescription drugs, demand tends to be inelastic. Compared with necessities, luxuries have a greater income (and price) elasticity of demand. That is, a decrease in income (or an increase in price) is assumed to generate a greater decline in the demand for luxuries than the demand for necessities. The more money spent on luxury items, the less income left for attaining necessities and securing the future. In contrast, spending income or money on necessities has an ultimate justification: one just cannot do without them.

Elasticity changes over time. Habit and existing commitments limit the extent to which consumers can respond to price changes in the short run. This is a form of gradual adaptation to loss, and learning. For example, when gas prices increase, consumers typically initially balk at gas prices they consider outrageous, but then after a period of weeks or months, they readjust their opinion on what is expensive.

Pricing Decision

The price elasticity of demand is a basic building block in making a pricing decision. For example, convenience stores have much higher markup on specialty or emergency items, such as deli food or cold remedies, than on everyday items, such as milk or soft drinks that can be bought anywhere. In general, markups are higher when demand is less elastic than when it is more elastic.

Charging according to what the market will bear is referred to as *price discrimination*. In economics, price discrimination occurs when prices for the same product are observed to differ without any clear differences in the costs of production or distribution. Price discrimination leads to different prices paid by different buyers. For example, airlines charge higher prices for first-class seating and lower prices for advance purchase. Movie theaters charge lower prices for matinees and for senior citizens. Each of these industries is pricing according to these different groups' willingness to pay; each group has a different price-quantity relationship.

In a slow economy, most products go on sale; however, some products remain untouched by discounts. One reason is *consumer habit formation*— old habits die hard. For example, customers may see discounts for food and clothing, but not for tobacco products. This is because most smokers will not switch from the brand they currently use (brand loyalty), and instead they will cut their spending in other areas. Also, many retailers tend to resist markdowns because lower prices can threaten a brand's well-cultivated image. For example, discounts are infrequent in stores like Abercrombie & Fitch and Apple. This is in part a reaction to consumers' *conspicuous consumption*: consumption as driven in part by a desire to project a favorable image and to achieve social status. Retail stores are careful not to set a precedent that gets consumers accustomed to huge markdowns, making them less willing to spend on full-price products.

CONCLUSION

Problems of scarcity are the basis for the development and use of the economist's tools and criteria. Every decision to use resources, therefore, has an opportunity cost in that those resources cannot be used to produce benefits elsewhere. The traditional economic perspective relies on a "market" approach in which suppliers compete for customers on the basis of price and quality. The market mechanisms are believed the most effective mechanisms for allocating resources. Standard economics assumes that we are rational—that we set goals and pursue them intelligently by using the information and resources at our disposal, and that we are cognitively able in weighing the consequences of each potential option. Behavioral economics has recognized that the rational choice model is inaccurate in some systematic and important ways, and that to take full advantage of the economic insights and methodology, economists must embrace insights from psychology and other social sciences so as to make economics more relevant and realistic. Behavioral economics attempts to understand these departures and, more generally, integrate psychologists' understanding of human behavior into economic analysis.

4

An Economic Perspective on Eating Behavior

INTRODUCTION

The economic framework discussed in Chapter 3 provides another explanation for the observed links between economic variables and eating behavior. Chapter 2 demonstrated that the rapid growth of obesity in the United States over the past few decades is better explained by behavior rather than genes. The economic view suggests that behavior is affected by economic incentives. This chapter provides an economic perspective on overeating resulting from the decreased price of foods and other economic factors, such as technologic advances, consumer lifestyle choice, and time pressure. These factors provide key policy tools for promoting dietary change.

THE ECONOMICS OF FOOD CONSUMPTION DECISIONS

As explained in the previous chapter, one of the goals of economics is to understand how people decide to allocate their limited resources (e.g., money, time, efforts) among available alternatives. A central assumption in economics is the notion that individuals seek to maximize total utility (i.e., their happiness), that is, choose the option that will yield the greatest utility, given the constraints imposed by available resources. The concept of utility refers to how desirable a choice is for an individual. By definition, people pursue whatever behavior has the highest utility.

Consumers choose foods based on taste (palatability), price, convenience, and health. Food choice presents a conflict between the satisfaction of appetites (immediate desires) and the consequences for physical appearance and health (delayed rewards). One can satisfy nutritional requirements at a low cost by selecting certain foods, such as liver, dry legumes, peanuts, and canned fish, but for many people, such a diet may also be low in taste. Food price also influences choice. For example, given a choice of two alternative foods, such as snack foods (A) and fruits and vegetables (B), the choice of A depends on both the price and the preference of consuming A relative to B. As the price of B increases, consumers may shift their choice to A. It is well established that the diets of lower-income persons consist of cheap foods, since healthier diets cost more (Drewnowski & Darmon, 2005). Obese and overweight individuals may have higher preferences for snack foods relative to fruits and vegetables.

Consumers face two constraints: total calories and budgetary constraint. Given those two constraints, each person's food choices are designed to maximize direct benefits associated with food consumption. The economic rule for optimal allocation decision calls for equality at the margin. This means relating the marginal utility (benefit) to the incremental cost of consumption. In other words, consumption continues for as long as the marginal benefit of the next unit consumed is equal to or greater than its marginal cost. The marginal benefit can take the form of reduced hunger, satisfaction, or sheer enjoyment. Although positive, it diminishes as more food is consumed. The two components of marginal cost are food price and the negative impact of any additional consumption on the utility of food. For example, the observation that energy-dense foods are highly palatable suggests that the marginal benefits of consuming these foods are high. The observation that the same foods provide dietary energy at a very low cost suggests that the marginal cost of consuming additional units is low.

From an economic perspective, maximizing utility means that consumer food choice is not determined solely by good health but utility, in which good health is only one factor. Rational persons constantly trade-off health for competing goods, such as taste and time (convenience). For example, among low-income households or the unemployed attempting to maintain food costs, it is taste and cost that are the key determinants of food choice. So, low-income families will place higher priority on energy-dense foods in order to allocate their limited resources on other items, such as rent and clothing (Drewnowski, 1997). Thus, food costs may represent a barrier to choosing healthy foods.

Price

Price defined broadly (including monetary, time, and health consequences) is a powerful influence. A basic principle of economics is that increasing the price of a commodity reduces purchases. When food is abundant and cheap, people will eat more of it and gain weight. Economic studies conclude that falling food prices may be one of the primary reasons for the rising obesity problem. Philipson and Posner (1999) report that about 40% of weight growth in the 1980s and 1990s seems to be due to a drop in real food prices[1] through technological innovation

---

[1]Real prices are expressed in constant dollars and usually reflect buying power relative to a base year. Real price is adjusted to remove the effect of changes in the purchasing power of the dollar.

in agriculture. Cutler, Glaeser, and Shapiro (2003) show that the general prices of snacks and food from vending machines have declined; thus increasing caloric intake obtained through snacking over time. On the other hand, the fruit and vegetable price index has risen in real terms in recent years. Low relative prices may explain why lower-income households tend to choose diets high in refined grains and added sugar and fats (Drewnowski & Darmon, 2005).

Price elasticity[2] for foods and nonalcoholic beverages ranges from 0.27 to 0.81 (absolute values). Soft drinks, juice, and meats have higher elasticity (0.7–0.8). On the other hand, oils (0.48), sugars and sweets (0.34), and eggs (0.27) are most inelastic (Andreyeva, Long, & Brownell, 2009). For example, a 10% increase in soft drink prices should reduce consumption by about 8%. It is important to note that these estimates are for food categories. Elasticity for specific types of food (e.g., a specific type of apple) tend be higher as a result of availability of more substitutes. From a policy perspective, foods with larger price elasticity should be targeted to change consumer consumption behaviors, such as encouraging people to increase their consumption of fruits and vegetables in response to a price decline.

Studies show that the relative price of different products has more potent effect on food choice than nutritional labeling. Simone French et al. (2001) manipulated the prices of high-fat and low-fat snacks in vending machines at 12 high schools and 12 workplaces. In some cases, the snacks were labeled to indicate their fat content. The results showed that the price changes, rather than the labels, had significant effect on purchase. Dropping the price of the low-fat snacks by even a nickel spurred more sales. Reducing the price of low-fat snack foods by 10%, 25%, and 50% was associated with sales increases of 9%, 39%, and 93%, respectively. In contrast, orange stickers signaling low-fat content or cartoons promoting the low-fat alternatives had little influence over which snacks were more popular. Average profits per machine were not affected by the vending interventions. The findings suggest that reducing the prices of low-fat snack food consistently increased the purchase of those items.

---

[2]In economics, the own price elasticity of demand measures the responsiveness of quantity demanded to changes in price. It is a measure of how sensitive the quantity demanded is to a change in the price of the good. When the relative change in purchased quantity is greater than the relative change in price, demand is elastic (the absolute value price elasticity is more than 1). If changes in quantity demanded is below the relative change in price, demand is inelastic (the absolute value price elasticity is less than 1). For example, when a commodity purchased quantity falls by 3.2% due to a 10% increase in price, the price elasticity of demand is -0.32, reflecting inelastic demand. Elasticity is determined by the number of substitutes, consumer income, expected duration of price change, and the product market share. For example, products with fewer substitutes generally have a lower elasticity, and hence are price-inelastic.

Evidence shows that the price of fast food is negatively related to body weight among adolescents, whereas the price of fruits and vegetables is positively related to body weight. For example, Chou, Grossman, and Saffer (2004) find that food prices in fast-food and full-service restaurants and in grocery stores are all negatively correlated with individuals' BMI. Goldman, Lakdawalla, and Zheng (2009) estimated that in the short run, a 10% price reduction would lead to a BMI increase of 0.22 units (or 0.6%). But, in the long run (30 years), the price reduction will lead to a BMI increase of 1.5 units (or 3.6%). Sturm and Datar (2008) shows that the effect of food prices on body weight among children became larger during a 5-year period. The findings suggest that taxes on fast food would have to be substantial in order to have any meaningful effect on weight. On the other hand, Powell et al. (2009) found that young adults' fruit and vegetable consumption levels were significantly associated with prices, with an estimated price elasticity of consumption of −0.32. This means that the demand for fruits and vegetables is inelastic. This suggests that subsides or reducing taxes on fruits and vegetables are likely to promote healthy eating, especially among lower income and young adults.

Time Scarcity and Food Choice

The full "price" of food also includes the value of time spent acquiring, preparing, cooking, and cleaning up after meals. An economic perspective on time describes people as rational individuals who seek to maximize utility. The household is like a small firm that produces basic goods (meals, entertainment) through a combination of market goods and services (food ingredients), resources (cooking equipment and skills), and time (food preparation). As time becomes more precious, people naturally spend less time on food preparation. They tend to substitute calorie-dense fast food for more healthful home-cooked meals. The main point of the economic perspective is recognizing and valuing time as a resource and constraint in producing and consuming goods and services. With limited time, many consumers choose takeout or foods prepared outside the home.

Time scarcity, the feeling of not having enough time, contributes to food choices such as a decrease in food preparation at home and an increase in the consumption of convenience or ready-prepared foods. These food choices are associated with less nutritional quality and may contribute to obesity. People report less time preparing and eating meals at home due to busy schedules. In 2001, 72% of U.S. married couples with children 18 years of age or younger were employed compared with 47% in 1975 (Ramey, 2009). In 1900, women accounted for 21% of the labor force and married women for less than 6%, but by 1999, women—married or not—accounted for more than 60% (Ramey, 2009). Working women were unable or unwilling to spend as much time grocery shopping, cooking, and cleaning up after meals (Ramey, 2009).[3] Chou et al. (2004) report that growth in the price of women's time has made it more costly to monitor the intake of calories at home and has led to growth in the demand for unhealthy fast food. They show that the rise in average hours worked by mothers can account for as much as one-third of the growth in obesity among children in certain families. As more women and men work outside the home, they have less time to supervise the activities of their children. Reduced parental supervision may be associated with watching more TV, snacking, and less participation in recreational activities.

Many of the market-driven changes to the current U.S. food distribution system have reduced the time required to procure and prepare food by providing convenient, ready-to-eat snack foods, microwavable meals, vending machines at workplaces and schools, and drive-through windows at fast-food restaurants. These changes may have inadvertently made the environment more food-friendly for consumers. It is extremely easy to access large quantities of food and expend hardly any time or energy doing so (Bowers, 2000).

Cutler et al. (2003) show that technological innovation has reduced the time costs of food preparation. Lowering the time needed to acquire and prepare food increases the frequency of eating and shifts diets toward convenience foods, which tend to be more caloric. While the price reduction affects all, the reduced time delay will mostly affect individuals with self-control problems.

Shift to Eating Out

Eating out has become a way of life for many American families. As time becomes more precious, people naturally spend less time on food preparation—substituting calorie-dense fast food for more healthful home-cooked meals. And because incomes have risen, people can afford to eat out more often. The average American spends less than 10% of his or her income for food (Engel's law)[4] (Drewnowski, 1997).

USDA food-intake surveys indicate that Americans increased the share of daily caloric intake from food away from home from 18% to 32%

---

[3]Bowers, D. E. Cooking trends echo changing roles of women. FoodReview, 2000;23(1): 23–29.

[4]Engel's law states that as incomes increase, the proportion of income spent on food falls. In 2006, U.S. households spent a smaller percentage of their income on food than households in any other country (7.2%). By contrast, the figure was 22% in Poland and more than 40% in Egypt and Vietnam.

between the late 1970s and mid-1990s. In 2007, about a third of the population consumed at least one meal a day away from home, and an estimated 42% of every food dollar was spent on food prepared by others, up from 25% in 1970 (Clauson & Leibtag, 2008).

Data from the Census of Retail Trade (Christian & Rashad, 2009) highlight the steady increase in the number of full-service and fast-food restaurants since the early 1970s; between 1972 and 1997, the number of restaurants per 10,000 population increased by 61% from 884 to 1427. Chou et al. (2004) present findings that the state-level growth in availability of restaurants accounts for the majority of the growth in weight over time. However, the causality may run on the opposite direction. That is, the growth in the number of restaurants is driven by consumer preferences and food choices.

Individuals who consume more of their food away from home are more likely to consume meals lower in nutritional quality and higher in caloric intakes. Food consumed away from home is higher in total fat and lower in dietary fiber, calcium, and iron (Guthrie, Lin, & Frazao, 2002). Home cooks and restaurants have different incentives with regard to caloric supply. The home cook presumably internalizes the health costs of a calorically rich diet; the restaurateur does not. Hence, the latter will have a greater incentive to supply food that creates addictive cravings (such as sweets). Manufacturers of food have invested heavily in making their products tastier, cheaper, more varied, and more convenient for the consumer. This suggests that increasing information on calorie and nutrition content could help people to make better healthful choices.

Food Cost and Availability

The greater efficiency, specialization, and size of the American food system have produced plentiful and cheaper food. More and more food is being produced by fewer people and with less capital. For example, the average daily calories available in the U.S. food supply increased by more than 500 calories per person between 1970 and 2004 (Shapouri & Rosen, 2008). The U.S. food supply—plus imports less exports—provides a daily average of 3,900 calories per capita (Shapouri & Rosen, 2008). This level is nearly twice the amount needed to meet the energy requirements of most people. Marion Nestle (2002) argues that this overabundance alone is sufficient to explain why food companies compete so strenuously for consumer food dollars.

One result of overabundance is pressure to add value to foods through processing. The transformation of raw commodities into finished goods is known as *adding value*. For example, the conversion of potatoes (cheap) to potato chips (expensive) fried in artificial fats or coated in soybean flour or herbal supplement is an example of how value is added to basic food commodities.

At the end of the process, the initial cost of the raw material is only a tiny fraction of the retail price. The producers of raw foods receive only a fraction of the price that consumers pay at the supermarket. For example, of the $3.25 price of 12-ounce box of cereal at the supermarket, less than 25 cents represent the cost of the grain itself. Heavily processed products offer the highest potential markups. For example, soft drink sold in chain restaurants are little more than syrup and carbonated tap water, the can provides a profit margin of about 90% (Kessler, 2009).

The farm value share of the retail price of food (based on prices farmers receive for commodities) has been used to determine how processed certain foods are. In 1998, for example, an average of 20% of retail cost—the "farm value" of the food—was returned to its producers (Nestle, 2002). The remaining 80% of the food dollars goes for labor, packaging, advertising, and other such value-enhancing activities. Overall, the farm value share of the retail price of food has declined from 41% in 1950 to an estimated 19% in 2006. The percentage of farm value, however, is unequally distributed. Opportunities for adding value to fresh fruits and vegetables are limited, and thus they have little potential for markup (Dunham, 1994).

Substitution and Complements

Eating represents a choice among many alternative food selections. Individual choice depends on the rewarding value and prices of those alternatives. If the price of an alternative is increased, then consumer will shift choice from preferred to less-preferred foods. The alternative commodity is called a substitute (e.g., for some consumers, tea may be a substitute for coffee). Food items also may have complementary relationships (e.g., for some consumers, mustard is a complement to hot dogs). In a complementary relationship, when price for a commodity increases, the consumption of a complement commodity decreases. For example, TV watching is associated with poor dietary habits, and reducing television watching can reduce food intake. Similarly, for many people, socializing and eating are complements. Since the early 1980s, there has been a decrease in relative prices of calorie-dense foods and drinks relative to fruits and vegetables (Finkelstein, Ruhm, & Kasa, 2005). As unhealthy food became relatively cheaper, people substituted away from healthy food toward unhealthy food.[5]

---

[5]Several factors explain why healthy foods are expensive, such as higher costs of transportation, refrigeration, labor, and packaging, and being prone to spoilage.

The concept of substitution has important implications for eating behavior. For example, consider the choice between social interactions with friends and food. Overweight youths are more likely to eat than engage in social interactions with peers (Epstein et al., 2008). Inadequate social skills may increase the price of social interaction and encourage overweight youth to substitute easily accessible pleasurable foods. Moreover, the desirability of eating a particular food may increase with repeated consumption over time, which may lead to excessive appetite for the food, and reducing the ability to seek alternative behavior. Thus, building strong friendship and social supports for children could lead to substituting social interaction for eating.

The concept of substitution explains why people tend to gain weight after quitting smoking. The percentage of adults who smoked regularly dropped from 42.4% in 1965 to 20.9% in 2004. Economic studies have shown that higher cigarette taxes and higher cigarette prices cause more smokers to quit, but these smokers seem to start eating more as a result (Chou et al., 2004). A 10% increase in the real price of cigarettes produces a 2% increase in the number of obese people, other things being equal (Chou et al., 2004). The inflation-adjusted price of cigarettes has risen by approximately 164% since 1980. This increase accounts for almost 20% of the growth in obesity after 1980.[6] Of course, this is not to suggest that antismoking campaigns are a mistake, and people should start smoking in order to become thin, substituting one type of unhealthy behavior for another.[7] Clearly, those who curtail their habit or quit smoking altogether typically gain weight as the appetite-suppressing and metabolism-increasing effects of smoking come to an end. Smoking dulls one's taste buds, meaning that food becomes less appealing.[8] Also, smokers attempting to quit may feel the need to put something in their mouths to replace cigarettes ("oral fixation").

---

[6]The effect of cigarette smoking on obesity remains inconclusive. These conflicting results have been attributed to differences in methods of investigation. For example, a recent study reports that in the long run, a rise in cigarette prices is actually associated with a decrease in both BMI and obesity using the different method (Courtemanche, 2009). When a person overcomes the smoking addiction, he/she may gain confidence in his/her ability to develop healthier habits.

[7]Since more Americans are obese than who smoke, some experts fear that antismoking campaigns could have actually worsened public health.

[8]This explains why adolescent females sometimes use smoking as a method of weight control.

THE EFFECT OF FAST FOODS ON OBESITY

How do changes in the supply of fast-food restaurants affect eating behavior? Public health experts argue that the widespread availability of fast-food restaurants is an important contributor to obesity. For example, the presence of a fast-food restaurant within a 10th of a mile of a school was associated with an increase of about 5.2% increase in incidence of obesity among 9th grade children (Currie, Vigna, Moretti, & Pathania, 2009).[9] However, there may be a reverse causality between fast food and demand for unhealthy foods. Fast food chains are likely to open new restaurants where they expect demand to be strong. In other words, fast-food chains did not create our craving for fats, sugar, and salt, they merely exploited a taste already well established.

Proximity to fast-food restaurants simply leads to substitution away from food prepared at home or consumed in other restaurants. The proximity to fast food could lower the money and time price of accessing unhealthy food. In addition, the proximity may increase consumption by tempting those consumers with self-control problems. A fast-food restaurant in immediate proximity is more likely to trigger a cue that leads to increase in demand. The policy implication is that limiting access to fast food could have a beneficial impact on populations with limited ability to travel, such as school children.

FOOD MARKETING

Food marketing refers to any activity conducted by a company in the food, beverage, or restaurant industry to encourage purchase of its products. As noted in Chapter 2, food preferences develop at a very early age, primarily through learning processes. Once established, these eating patterns are difficult to change. Parents are a key influence in the early development of food preferences; however, outside influences become increasingly important, especially during middle childhood and adolescence (Institute of Medicine [IOM], 2006). Food marketing promotes highly desirable, but unhealthy, products to youth. The overexposure to food marketing presents a public health issue to youth (Harris, Brownell, & Bargh, 2009). Unlike tobacco and alcohol consumption, young people do not need to learn that consuming these foods is rewarding. From birth, humans prefer the taste of foods high in sugar, fat, and salt (i.e., the foods most commonly advertised).

---

[9] http://emlab.berkeley.edu/~moretti/obesity.pdf

The rise in childhood obesity has raised concerns that food marketing contributes to unhealthy food preferences and eating behaviors (IOM, 2006). Over one-third of children and adolescents in the United States are overweight or at risk for becoming overweight, and the rate more than tripled from 1971 to 2004. Public health experts believe that the food environment is a leading cause of this obesity epidemic, due in part to the overwhelming number of marketing messages that encourage consumption of calorie-dense food products of low nutritional value (IOM, 2006). Moreover, children are less likely to have information about the consequences of their action or to heavily discount these consequences.

Food companies in the United States spend huge amounts (e.g., $1.6 billion in 2006) (IOM, 2006) in marketing to youth, especially young children, to increase the demand for their goods. In 2004, the average child in the United States viewed approximately 15 television food advertisements every day (IOM, 2006). Nearly all of these advertisements (98%) promote products (high in sugar, fat, and/or sodium) that young people should only consume in very limited quantities (IOM, 2006). In contrast, public service announcements represent only 0.8% of nonprogramming content viewed by children on television (IOM, 2006). Thus, marketing of unhealthy foods designed to taste great poses an unfair advantage over marketing and education to promote healthy foods (e.g., "5-a-day" fruit and vegetable programs).

From an economic perspective, the purpose of advertising is for a firm to increase its demand. Economists have developed three conceptual views as to why consumers respond to advertising (Bagwell, 2005). The first view is that advertising is persuasive. This view suggests that advertising alters consumers' tastes and encourages brand loyalty through product differentiation (or product reputation). As a consequence, the demand for a firm's product becomes more inelastic.

The second view is that advertising is informative. In this view, advertising provides a useful role by providing information to consumers,[10]

---

[10]Products can be classified based on their pre-purchased characteristics, such as search, experience, and credence. Search goods are those that a buyer can readily evaluate prior to purchase by observation—style of a dress or simple test of a food item. Experience goods are those that a buyer can evaluate only after consuming the product. The buyer, therefore, does not know exactly what he or she is getting the first time he or she buys it (e.g., the taste of a packaged food or the effectiveness of a dishwashing detergent). Advertising is especially important for experience goods. Goods with credence attributes are those that a buyer cannot confidently evaluate even after one purchase. Consumers, therefore, must rely heavily on the product's reputation with respect to those attributes, even for repeat purchases. A buyer normally cannot, for example, evaluate a doctor's competence after one visit for the treatment of one complaint. In the case of food, for example, credence attributes characterize organic food products. Public policy plays an important role for goods with credence attributes in protecting consumers (e.g., food safety standards and accurate labeling).

which results in more competition and increased elasticity of the demand for a firm's product. According to the informative view, observed price dispersion in the market can be interpreted as a reflection of consumer ignorance. The ignorance reflects the consumers' search costs of obtaining information as to the existence, location, and prices of products.

The third view is that advertising is complementary to the advertised product, and serves to increase the demand for the product. Consumers may simply derive more satisfaction (utility) from consuming a more advertised good. For example, consumers may value "social prestige," and the consumption of a product may generate greater prestige when the product is advertised.

Marketing can be distinguished between *informational marketing* (that provides rational benefits and reasons to purchase or consume a product) and *emotional marketing* (messages designed to simply make the consumer feel good about the product). Economics treats advertising as a cognitive process. In this approach, individuals must actively process information presented before attitude change can occur.[11]

Food marketing is primarily emotional. Emotional marketing is designed to influence consumer decision making through unconscious, or automatic, processes, and to develop strong emotional connections between consumers and brands from a very early age through high levels of advertising directed toward young consumers. Positive emotions toward advertisements translate to positive brand evaluations and behavior intentions. Later on, this positive response becomes a source of information, or *heuristic*, for brand evaluation (e.g., Schwarz & Clore, 1988). For example, repeated brand exposure will increase liking of the brand through mere exposure effects. This suggests that the earlier children are exposed to food advertising messages, the more susceptible they may be to long-lasting effects.

Television advertising communicates positive outcomes (such as happiness, or being "cool" with no negative consequences) from consuming nutrient-poor foods. Food marketing rarely conveys the consequences of unhealthy eating, including weight gain, low energy levels, or long-term health effects. Moreover, food advertising typically focuses on the immediate sensory gratifications of consumption (i.e., the "hot" appetitive features), making resistance to these messages even more difficult (i.e., the "cold," rational process of self-restraint). In other words,

---

[11]Research shows that, before the age of 7 or 8 years, children do not have the cognitive capacity to understand that advertising presents a biased point of view. Numerous studies show that before the age of 8 years, most children believe that advertising is intended simply to provide them with information, and they are much more likely to believe that commercials always tell the truth.

snack ads encourage a short-term hedonic enjoyment goal, whereas nutrition ads encourage a long-term goal of healthy eating. Food marketing attempts to differentiate comparable brands by establishing positive brand responses. The distinction between Coke and Pepsi provide a classic example of the power of emotional advertising. In a blind taste test, researchers find that subjects split equally in their preferences for Coke and Pepsi (McClure, Laibson, Loewenstein, & Cohen, 2004). However, when one cup was labeled "Coke," individuals (coke drinkers) showed a strong emotional attachment to the brand at the neurological level (McClure et al., 2004). When the subjects were informed that they were drinking Coke, brain regions associated with memory were activated. *Expectancy theory* provides a potential mechanism to explain[12] this finding. The theory suggests that expectancies about a food influence individuals' actual taste experience. For example, preschoolers liked the taste of foods and beverages significantly more when they were placed in McDonald's packaging, compared with the same foods in plain packaging (Harris et al., 2009). Furthermore, repeated exposure to food advertising can affect food preferences through its influence on normative beliefs.

Young people (as well as adults) may find it difficult to believe that they are affected outside of their conscious awareness, and far more developed cognitive abilities may be required to defend against automatic influences as compared with more direct persuasive attempts. In addition, defending against the massive number of subtle marketing messages encountered daily may be extraordinarily difficult. According to one estimate, consumers see 3,000 marketing messages daily (Harris et al., 2009). If this process takes as little as 10 seconds, defending against marketing messages would require 8 hours out of every day. Furthermore, resisting the influence of tempting images of highly desirable foods requires self-regulatory resources, which can become depleted in the short-term, especially under conditions of fatigue (Baumeister, Heatherton, & Tice, 1994). Thus, food advertising may have a greater influence on both children and adults, for example, when watching television to unwind at the end of a long day.

In sum, the psychological models of marketing suggest that the effects of food marketing exposure may be difficult to counteract. Youth marketing is powerfully effective, occurs in massive amounts, and is done in forms that thwart cognitive defenses and subvert parents' ability to monitor what their children see and ultimately their ability to provide their children with a healthy food environment. Recent pledges by the food industry in the United States to reduce unhealthy marketing to children,

---

[12]Mechanisms refer to psychological processes through which exposure to an external stimulus causes behavior.

as well as a recent (2008) ban on junk food advertising to children in the United Kingdom, clearly suggest that companies believe they must respond to public perceptions about negative effects of food marketing. The knowledge of the psychological mechanisms that increase preference and consumption of unhealthy foods suggests increased awareness and understanding of how unwanted external influences might affect us. This body of work highlights the need for media literacy programs and the public understanding of how advertising may affect them outside of their awareness.

SOCIAL COSTS

Obesity has created social as well as private costs. For example, there is a strong positive correlation between BMI and Type 2 diabetes. Overweight and obesity have become to diabetes what tobacco is to lung cancer. A national survey in 2007 (Hu, 2008) found that 85% of diabetics were overweight or obese.[13] Obese adults have about 10 times the risk of developing diabetes compared with normal-weight adults (Hu, 2008). Insulin resistance is often considered the common mechanism underlying the clustering of multiple metabolic disorders related to obesity.[14] It is estimated that over 90% of diabetes is attributable to unhealthy diet and lifestyle (Hu, 2008). Also, the risks increase as we age. According to the Centers for Disease Control and Prevention, one in 10 Americans has diabetes (24 million people), and if present trends continue, one in three will suffer from the disease by the year 2050 (Flegal, Carroll, Ogden, & Curtin, 2010). The cost for the health care system is $174 billion a year (Flegal et al., 2010). Diabetes patients spend an average of $6000 annually for treatment of their disease, such as monitoring supplies, medicines, doctor

---

[13]Diabetes results when the body cannot use blood sugar as energy, either because it has too little insulin or because it cannot use insulin. In diabetes, the body either produces too little insulin (Type 1) or is resistant to insulin (Type 2), causing excess levels of glucose in the blood. Type 2 (non–insulin-dependent) diabetes accounts for 90% to 95% of all cases of diabetes. This form of diabetes, which used to develop so exclusively in adulthood, is now increasingly seen in children.

[14]Obesity triggers a plethora of metabolic disturbances, including insulin resistance, hypertension, hyperglycemia, hypertriglyceridemia, and reduced levels of high-density lipoprotein (HDL), together referred to as the metabolic syndrome. The World Health Organization defined metabolic syndrome as insulin resistance and/or impaired glucose regulation with at least three or more of the following conditions: abdominal obesity (waist circumference > 40 inches. in men and >35 inches. in women; hypertriglyceridemia $\geq$ 150 mg/dL; low HDL cholesterol < 40 mg/dL in men and <50 mg/dL in women; high blood pressure $\geq$ 130/85 mm Hg; and high fasting glucose $\geq$ 110 mg/dL. Approximately, one quarter of U.S. adults (or 47 million people) have the metabolic syndrome.

visits, and annual eye exams (Finkelstein, Trogdon, Cohen, & Dietz, 2009). The inability to shoulder this high cost, in part, explains why only 25% of diabetics are getting the care they need (Finkelstein et al., 2009).

More generally, it is estimated that the obesity-related medical spending explains 27% of the growth in real health care spending from 1987 to 2001 (Thorpe, Florence, Howard, & Joski, 2004).The evidence from developed countries is that high BMI is associated with greater absenteeism at work and at school due to health (Geier et al., 2007). Early obesity strongly predicts later cardiovascular disease.

Overweight individuals are the target of prejudice and discrimination (Puhl & Brownell, 2001). Many people believe that a lack of willpower is to blame for the obesity epidemic. Overall, obese individuals are perceived as less intelligent, less hardworking, less attractive, less popular, less successful, less athletic, and more weak willed than are individuals with normal weight (Hebl & Mannix, 2003). Individuals suffering from obesity are stigmatized in part by the belief that the decision to overeat is completely under voluntary control. People tend to equate body size with Puritan values. Thin means self-discipline and hard work; fat implies laziness, gluttony, and lack of willpower. Being overweight—especially among women—is strongly stigmatized in our society, and often leads to reactive depression and social isolation. Puhl and Brownell (2001) examined discrimination toward obese people in the areas of employment, education, and health care. They found that 28% of teachers believed that becoming obese is the worst thing that can happen to a person; 24% of nurses felt repulsed by obese persons; and parents provided less college support for their overweight children than for their thin children. Discrimination also reduces obese women's marriage prospects (Gortmaker, Must, Perrin, Sobol, & Dietz, 1993). The available evidence shows that obesity reduces dating opportunities, and the effect is more stringent for females. Surveys of college students show that they (especially boys) prefer to date thinner partners (Cawley, 2004).

Stigmatization and discrimination lead to lower earnings for the obese. Recent evidence shows that obese men suffer a 5% wage penalty, whereas obese women on average make 12% less than their normal-weight counterparts (Cawley, 2004; Mocan & Tekin, 2009). Obesity or overweight may impact wages through different mechanisms (Cawley, 2004). First, in some occupations, obesity may have a direct detrimental impact on labor productivity. Second, obesity may cause discrimination by employers or customers. Third, obesity may lower productivity through its impact on poor health, and the lower wages reflect the higher health care costs. Finally, obesity may lower wages through lower self-esteem. Physically attractive workers are more confident, which impacts their wages positively.

In light of this pervasive prejudice against individuals who are overweight and obese, it is no surprise that being obese is associated with increased levels of depression and with decreased levels of self-esteem. However, as obesity begins to rise, the negative image of obesity becomes less intense because obesity is now more common. This further helps obesity continue to grow.

THE ECONOMIC RATIONALE FOR PUBLIC POLICY

In economic terms, *negative externalities* arise when obesity generates costs for nonobese persons. The behavior is a form of *moral hazard*,[15] meaning that individual members of society have less incentive to engage in behavioral change. If individuals do not bear all the costs of their decisions, then government interventions may improve social welfare. Thus, public policies modifying such unhealthy habits are very important. This section describes several rationales for public interventions.

A *market failure* occurs when the market fails to provide the necessary incentives for an individual to make a decision that will impact others not directly involved in the decision. Market failures have been identified and discussed in the literature on obesity in the following three areas: limited information, externalities, and lack of rationality.

First, it is possible that people make unhealthy choices because they are poorly informed. There may be lack of information regarding what constitutes healthy habits and, more specifically, the calorie content of purchased foods. Information about the calorie content of purchased food may be insufficient, or costly to obtain.

Second, the obese incur higher lifetime costs than the nonobese. Obesity accounts for 9.1% of all medical spending, about $147 billion in 2008, and it is blamed for about 112,000 premature deaths annually in the United States (Finkelstein et al., 2009). The annual medical expenditures of obese adults are 37% higher than expenditures of healthy weight individuals (Sturm, 2002). The health care consequences include 72 million people with a condition associated with diabetes, heart disease, some cancers, and other chronic illnesses (Finkelstein et al., 2009). In addition, obesity leads to a sicker workforce, which is a drag on economic growth (Cutler et al., 2003).[16] Externalities associated with obesity are likely to

---

[15]The tendency for insurance coverage to induce behavioral responses that raise the expected losses that are insured is called moral hazard.

[16]However, some studies suggest that the annual costs do not reflect the cumulative lifetime medical costs. Because obese people die younger and incur lower terminal medical costs than normal weight, their medical burden on society is neutral.

occur when health and life insurance premiums fail to consider that obese individuals tend to be sicker and have higher health care expenditures. In this case, some of the costs are borne by others or by society at large[17] (Bhattacharya & Sood, 2006).

Third, additional external effects may occur if individuals fail to recognize the impact of their choice of weight on their current and future well-being. This is known as *internality*, for instance, when individuals have self-control problems. Research indicate that a remarkably high proportion of individuals have self-control problems with respect to weight because they fail to stick to their self-declared weight-related plans. Individuals with self-control problems choose particular items based on the choice environment. This form of market failure has important implications for policy to influence choice environments that is conducive to increasing obesity. Policy makers would do well to consider a wide range of methods to tip people toward healthier food choices, including efforts to make healthy foods relatively cheaper or more convenient.

OBESITY PREVENTION POLICY

The followings describe examples of policies that have been introduced to counter obesity at the population level. All public health interventions can be classified as one of three broad categorical types of interventions: (1) education and information interventions, (2) incentives, and (3) laws and regulation. The information measures are aimed at correcting imperfect information to enable consumers to make better-informed choices. To correct market failures such as externalities, consumers are made to pay a price that reflect the true social cost of their actions (Mazzocchi, Traill, & Shogren, 2009). Policies on information measures constitutes the largest portion of the obesity prevention polices.

Education and Information Interventions

From an economic perspective, better information enables people to make informed choices, even though it may not improve their diets. Perfectly informed consumers choose their diets to maximize their own utility

---

[17]Under actuarial fairness, premiums would be set to equal expected health expenditures, and since those expenditures are potentially higher for the obese, premiums would also be higher for them. Generally, if risks differ in the population but individuals pay the same premium, this will create a positive subsidy for some individuals and a negative subsidy for others. The difference between lifetime expenditures and premium contributions gives the size of what is referred to as an insurance subsidy.

(satisfaction). They are informed about the health risks and the benefits of healthy eating. In economics, the welfare loss from poor information is referred to as the cost of ignorance. The key question is, to what extent the interventions promote healthier diets and improved health? Would the benefits exceed the costs?

More information on the diet-health relationships can lead to improved consumer choices. For example, with increasing coverage in the media about the risks Americans face if they continue their eating habits, millions of Americans are motivated to eat a more healthful diet. The U.S. Department of Agriculture (USDA) seized on this interest by designing a Web site, www.mypyramid.gov, that provides personalized eating guidelines. Users enter their age, sex, height, weight, and eating level and receive a table detailing their recommended daily intake in several food groups. Assessing the impact of information measures is complicated because the effects of public information policies are not immediate; it takes years for the health benefits to materialize. Moreover, people tend to forget information. Overall, studies indicate that information campaigns raise awareness but do not effectively change behavior (Mazzocchi et al., 2009).[18]

Nutrition labels are another primary source of information on food products. In the United States, nutrition labeling rules were set under the Nutritional Labeling and Education Act (NLEA), introduced in 1990. Nutrition labels typically include information on fat, saturated fat, sugar, salt, and calories. Do consumers make use of them in their purchasing decisions? Overall, evidence shows that consumers do make use of nutrition labels and they do have an impact on diet choices (Mazzocchi et al., 2009). Recent studies show a clear benefit to the subgroup of people motivated to improve their diet but with limited knowledge (Mazzocchi et al., 2009).[19] However, findings from the 2008 New York City's menu-labeling legislation (which made it mandatory for many restaurants to list calorie content on their menus) failed to show any effect on healthier eating. Lowenstein and colleagues examined purchases by 1,479 McDonald's customers in New York City in 2007 and 2008, both before and after menu labeling went into effect. Beyond simply measuring the impact of labeling, they gave some diners information about how many calories one is recommended to consume per day or per meal, anticipating that this information would

---

[18]An important obstacle to using nutritional labels is inadequate numeracy (comprehending labels). Rothman, Sheeran, Wood (2009) reports that only 32% of participants in a research study could accurately calculate the number of carbohydrates in a 20-oz soda with 2.5 servings.
[19]A British study suggests that "lower-fat" information for a meal in a restaurant was associated with it being chosen less frequently (Mazzocchi et al., 2009). Presumable, customers did not expect the low-fat meal to taste as good, and health was not a major factor in their decision of what to eat in a restaurant context.

help diners to make use of the posted calorie information. They found that this did not help diners use menu labels, and they saw no impact on calorie consumption.[20] It is interesting to note that labeling seems to attract more interest in avoiding "bad" nutrients than promoting "good" ones. For example, information on fats has an impact on consumer assessment of health risks, but information on fiber does not. This is consistent with the findings that negative information has a more powerful impact than positive information (Fox, Hayes, & Shogren, 2002).

The Effects of Food Marketing

Can advertising regulations, like banning junk food advertisements on children's TV programs, improve diet? The argument is that banning advertising would lead to less consumption of unhealthy foods. There is no longer a question about whether food marketing is hurting youth. The IOM (2006) report on children's food marketing sums up available knowledge in two words: "marketing works." Studies of food advertising show that time spent watching television was highly correlated with the unhealthy eating behaviors promoted in food advertising, preferences for unhealthy foods, and specific beliefs—for example, that fast food meals are as nutritious as meals prepared at home. In a longitudinal investigation, exposure to television, and therefore food advertising, in middle and high school predicted lower consumption of fruits, vegetables, and whole grains, as well as greater consumption of snack foods, fast food, and sugar-sweetened beverages 5 years later (Barr-Anderson, Larson, Nelson, Neumark-Sztainer, & Story, 2009).

Economists, as well, have found that exposure to fast food advertising increases adiposity in children, and estimate that banning fast food advertising would reduce the incidence of overweight children by 18% (Chou, Rashad, & Grossman, 2008).[21] An experimental study (Harris et al., 2009) found that lowering television viewing significantly reduced BMI in young children at or above the 75th BMI percentile, especially

---

[20]Requiring nutritional information in restaurants may be particularly beneficial for those who choose healthful foods. People who seek out and use calorie information are likely to be different from other eaters in many ways, including their motivation to cut calories. In other words, those who are intending to order lower-calorie meals are more likely to seek out the calorie information.

[21]These findings may be interpreted in support of the reverse causality. Media viewing may be explained by diet (children with low self-restraint may be more likely to watch television and consume unhealthy foods). Much of the relationship between television viewing and body mass index (BMI) could be due to increased food consumption while watching television.

for those in lower socioeconomic status households. The BMI reductions were due to reduced energy intake and not changes in physical activity.

Research among families in Quebec (where advertising to children under age 13 is banned) demonstrates that families purchase fast food less often than do similar families in Ontario (where there is no such ban) and that French-speaking families purchase less children's cereal than do English-speaking families (who watch television programming origi-nated primarily outside of Quebec) (Harris et al., 2009).

Market Intervention Measures

Economists have advocated direct policies to address the obesity exter-nality. These policies include taxes on unhealthy products (a "fat tax") and price support for health products. From an economic perspective, an important argument for the fat tax is that it internalizes the externalities associated with obesity. For example, a tax on soft drinks in Arkansas of about 2 cents per can generated revenues of $40 million per year (Mazzocchi et al., 2009). It is estimated that taxes on soft drinks and con-fectionary throughout the United States to generate about $1 billion per year (Mazzocchi et al., 2009). This money could be used to finance, for example, information policies.

However, tax policies may have unintended adverse effects on the poor; lower-income consumers tend to be more obese on average and eat more foods considered unhealthy (Brownell & Horgen, 2003). They are also more responsive to food prices—they have relatively higher price elasticity with respect to food. This implies that they would bear a greater share of the tax burden (Brownell & Horgen, 2003). An argument against the tax being regressive is the fact that obesity and diabetes affect the poor in greater numbers. Thus, the revenue from the tax could be targeted for helping the poor. Moreover, government taxation of less nutritious foods may be perceived as an infringement on civil liberties and personal choice, and be considered arbitrary, as it is difficult to uniformly classify foods as healthy or unhealthy.

The strongest and most consistent evidence (Smith, 2009) was ob-served for the effects of subsidizing healthy foods on increased purchases of those foods. This effect was large in terms of changes in food purchases and was observed across diverse settings (e.g., schools, worksites, restau-rants) and for various fruits and vegetables. In addition, total profits for vendors apparently were not reduced despite the price reduction. Even if subsidization increased the actual intake of healthy foods on a habit-ual basis, the question remains whether this would necessarily displace intake of unhealthy or energy-dense foods.

Farm Policy

Policymakers continue to debate the relationship between agricultural price support and diet. The issue is whether the subsidies to farmers lead to overproduction that encourages overconsumption of unhealthy foods, such as dairy products and sugar. Commodity crops, such as corn and soy, are processed into low-quality calories that make their way to consumers as refined starches, high-fructose corn syrup, hydrogenated oils, and feed for livestock. Kersh and Morone (2002) show that production of the nation's top three food sources of fat (i.e., red meat, plant oils, and dairy products) receive subsidies or other aid by federal, state, and/or local government.

Income Subsides

The US Food Stamp Program[22] has also been blamed for increased obesity rates, as recipients seem to consume more energy-dense foods than their noneligible counterparts (Smith, 2009). If assistance programs contribute to weight gain, then policy reform is required in ways that reduce this unintended consequence: for example, policies such as restricting the types of foods that can be purchased with food stamps, subsidizing recipients' purchase of healthy foods, offering cash instead of food stamps, and requiring recipients to take nutrition and health courses. Food stamps affect BMI through increased purchasing power and the monthly program cycle. Distributing higher or more frequent benefits might reduce disordered eating patterns and the associated weight gain (Smith, 2009). Offering discounts on healthy food, such as fresh produce and low-fat dairy products, might improve diets and BMI.

Food Availability at Schools

Concerns about childhood obesity have led people to call for restriction on the supply of unhealthy food made available to children at school. The main targets are school meals and vending machines that are loaded with unhealthy snacks and soft drinks. Restricting access to unhealthy options, such as the use of transfats or prohibiting soda and candy machines in

---

[22]What most people still call food stamps is technically the Supplemental Nutrition Assistance Program, or SNAP. In 2009, the program reached 36 million people. Virtually all have incomes near or below the federal poverty line (e.g., about $22,000 a year for a family of four). The Bush administration led a campaign to erase the program's stigma, calling food stamps "nutritional aid" instead of welfare, and made it easier to apply.

schools, is being tried across the country. Since 2005, 17 U.S. states have enacted legislation over vending machines in schools (Wansink, Just, & Payne, 2009). However, school administrators have argued against a ban on vending machines because they are reliant on the income to make up for shortfalls in school funding. In the United States, schools have contracts with fast food and soft drinks companies (e.g., 96% of schools had vending machines in 2000). A study at a county level found that financial pressure on schools is a good indicator of whether schools make junk foods available. Anderson and Butcher (2004) observed that a 10% increase in the proportion of schools in a county that make junk food available to their students is associated with a nearly 1% increase in students' BMI. This is particularly noticeable among those "vulnerable" (the increase among children with at least one obese parent was 2%).

CONCLUSION

This brief overview illuminates how a fairly standard economic framework can help explain some of the reasons behind food choices. Within the past several decades, several economic factors have tipped the balance between caloric intake and expense to an unfavorable equilibrium. These factors include growing quantity of caloric intake with declining overall food prices, rising costs of healthy foods relative to unhealthy foods, expanding labor market opportunities for women, and increased consumption of food away from home. Furthermore, technological innovations, such as vacuum packing, improved preservatives, and microwaves have made it possible to prepare food centrally with greater efficiency. The economic framework describes the importance of treating weight as a dynamic process that emphasizes the cumulative effects of economic incentives on body weight. The following chapters will add more realism to the economic perspective by incorporating the psychological and behavioral aspects of food consumption. In conclusion, it appears that public interventions that change the external factors (relative prices) are more effective than information measures in influencing consumer behavior. These policies are designed to make people responsible for the costs of their lifestyle decisions.

5

Socioeconomic Disparities in Health and Obesity

INTRODUCTION

Obesity does not occur randomly in populations. The rise in obesity is strongly related to socioeconomic disparities. This chapter focuses on the broader individual as well as social determinants of overweight and obesity. This approach is similar to the population health perspective. This perspective attempts to understand and explain obesity at the level of populations by going beyond the characteristics of the individual (e.g., diet, physical activity levels). This broader perspective on the determinants of obesity provides a useful complement to a physiological model of obesity, such as diet and physical activity. Understanding socioeconomic influences on obesity is important for effective prevention initiatives.

DEFINING SOCIOECONOMIC STATUS (SES)

Socioeconomic status (SES) has traditionally been defined by education, income, race, and rank (occupational status). These variables reflect one's status/position in the social hierarchy, wealth, and the associated social standing. SES is not a unified concept and consists of several dimensions. The SES indicators cannot be used interchangeably, since each indicator captures only a specific aspect of a person's socioeconomic circumstances over the life course. For instance, income is a measure of economic situation at one point of time, which is not sufficient to capture the long-term accumulation of economic resources, or the childhood economic situation. The whole spectrum of economic circumstances over the life course is expected to determine health status. Also, income is the indicator of the SES that can be most easily changed in the short term.

It is argued that addressing obesity requires closing the gap in income, education, and other factors influencing poverty (Marmot & Bell, 2009). Each SES indicator operates via a different mechanism to influence the development of obesity. Education influences knowledge and beliefs, occupation influences lifestyle, and income relates to access to health care resources. Alternatively, economic studies frequently focus on how health influences SES. Also, the SES-health correlation may be influenced by a "third factor." For instance, a high discount rate may be less willing to forgo current caloric intake for the future benefit of lower weight. In these cases, policies that improve health may boost access to economic resources.

Discounting of delayed rewards refers to the observation that the value of a delayed reward is considered to be worth less than an immediate reward. Higher discount rates give greater weight to benefits and costs accruing early in the life cycle than do lower discount rates. (For more discussion, see Chapter 6.)

HEALTH PRODUCTION FUNCTION

Economists study health status as a function of individuals' choices.[1] Some individuals are able to create and maintain healthy lifestyles. Most individuals place high value on their health and that of their family members. Economists assume the existence of a *"health production function"* that treats various socioeconomic variables as "input" and variables such as health status and children's height and test scores as "output." Socioeconomic variables such as maternal time allocation and household income affect intakes of energy and nutrition.

The health production function views health as a commodity that may be chosen like any other commodities subject to limited resources. Health inputs (lifestyle behaviors) are choices made by an individual as part of an attempt to achieve happiness over time. Individual choices involve trade-offs between future health or life expectancy and the immediate receipt of desirable nonhealthy goods. In many ways, individual lifestyle choices are fundamental to improvements in health status (McGinnis & Foege, 1993). Many major health problems in the United States and other developed nations, such as lung cancer, hypertension, and diabetes, are exacerbated by unhealthy behaviors. Lifestyle choices, such as tobacco use, overeating, and alcohol abuse, account for nearly one-third of all deaths in the United States (Cutler, Lleras-Muney, & Vogl, 2010). These behavioral choices dominate a person's health far more than the medical care system.

---

[1]In the same way, nutritionists study the effects of nutrients on health indicators based on biological science (simple associations). Nutrient intakes are inputs in a health production function.

Health Capital

Health is a form of capital.[2] From an economic perspective, health is treated as a durable-stock variable that depreciates with age and that can be improved by investing in health-producing activities, such as adopting a healthy diet. A key aspect of health capital is that health can be accumulated through education, lifestyle choices, and medical use. Investment[3] in health takes many forms. Immunization, annual checkups, exercise, and many other activities have current costs but may yield health benefits in the future.

Stock and Flow

Health capital, or *health stock*, is often measured by general levels of health or functioning, such as health status or the degree of difficulties with activities of daily living. Health flows describes the illness or morbidity conditions that an individual experiences over time. Healthy days are the benefits or services of that person's health capital or stock of health.

As mentioned, we can think about health as a durable good, much like an automobile, a home, or a child's education. We all come into the world with some inherent "stock" of health, some more than others. A normal healthy baby has a relatively high stock of health. Almost every action we take for the rest of our lives affects this stock of health. As with any durable good, our stock of health wears out over time. We call this process aging. As the stock of health falls low enough, we lose our ability to function and eventually die. Again, in economic terms, our stock of health depreciates. Death occurs when the stock of health falls below a life-sustaining level.

Life expectancy has increased dramatically during the past century, for example, implying that depreciation rate on people's stock of health has slowed through time. Public health efforts (such as sanitation, vaccination against communicable disease, etc.) and individual medical care all serve

---

[2]Similarly, cognitive capital, as a component of health capital, can be thought of as an asset that can be accumulated over time through education, work, and physical activities. The asset can be used throughout life to take advantage of opportunities and to maintain well-being in response to stress and other environmental challenges. Improving an individual's cognitive ability or reducing cognitive decline could have significant long-term health benefits, such as delaying dementia. When it comes to cognitive reserve, one must use it or lose it (Barnett, Salmond, Jones, & Sahakian, 2006).

[3]Broadly speaking, investment takes place when a tree is planted, when a student attends college, when you brush your teeth, as well as when you build a factory or a clinic. Any activity that can be expected to confer future benefits is a form of investment.

to slow down the rate of depreciation of health or to restore health to (or near) its original level after all illness or injury. Lifestyle choices such as exercise and proper nutrition (and smoking) are inputs that maintain or improve (or depreciate) one's stock of health. Similarly, body weight is a stock resulting from flows of caloric intake and expenditures.

Producing Health

The formulation of health production function (Grossman, 1972) begins with the idea that utility (happiness) is produced by health (H) and other goods (X). We can say that a person's utility function is of the form Utility = $U (X_1, H)$. The stock of health creates happiness. Our underlying desire for health itself leads us to desire lifestyle choices to help produce health. Our lifestyle choices, things we do and consume during our lives affect both the rate of aging and stock of health. Consumption of certain type of foods reduces our health. Since children and adolescents have the highest stock of health capital and the lowest rates of depreciation, they will be less likely than adults to choose a healthy diet. Similarly, the future would tend to be valued relatively less at old age. The expectation of a shorter and unhealthier life may discourage investment in human capital.

The model implies that individuals can value many things, not only health, and as a result, they may be willing to trade health for other things that they enjoy or value.[4] For example, a person might have full information about the consequences of smoking, but enjoy smoking so much that they are willing to accept worse health (and, therefore, surrender years of life) in exchange for the instantaneous pleasure of smoking.

The model also shows that every individual is both a demander and a producer of his own health. Specifically, individuals combine market goods and services with their own time to produce their health. The demand for health services like surgery or immunizations is a derived demand; people do not demand surgery because they enjoy it, they demand it because they value health and surgery is one way to increase their health. In short, the model considers "health" as an economic good and show how a rational person would have a demand for lifestyle choices "derived" from the underlying demand for health. The onset of poor health results in changes in time allocation as individuals experience

---

[4]In economic hard times, people respond by making trade-offs between necessities such as groceries, gas, housing, and medications (e.g., Lipitor cholesterol lowering medicine.) They may split pills or take their pills every other day. But they do not stop their pain medication because of the immediate negative effect. However, if enough people try to save money by forgoing drugs, controllable conditions could escalate into major medical problems that could eventually raise the nation's total health care costs.

illness. As the health capital falls, the amount of lost time increases, thereby reducing the amount of available time for health production.

Summary

Individuals choose a stream of health investments with the aim of maximizing lifetime happiness (utility). In making these choices, they are constrained both by what they know about the production of health capital and by their budgetary constraints. Healthy behaviors and disease detection is often cited as one solution to the aging population and the growing share of health care spending. Therefore, to the extent that individuals can be persuaded to consume effective preventative services today, their need for acute services in the future should be reduced. However, one significant barrier to adoption of preventive regimens is the fact that they generally require individuals to forgo consumption and activities that they enjoy today for the promise of some future payoff. The degree to which a person prefers the present relative to the future should therefore be an important determinant in their decisions with respect to the consumption of preventive services.[5]

SOCIOECONOMIC FACTORS AND HEALTH

This section provides a brief review of the associations between SES and health across the lifespan. Socioeconomic variables have fundamental influences on health and diseases. The health of populations is related to features of society and its social and economic organizations. These factors include SES, psychosocial characteristics, and social environment. On average, within developed countries, those lowest on the SES scale exhibit the poorest health, compared with those in the middle and those at the top (Marmot, 2006). For example, a 20-year-old low-income male, on average, reports to be in similar health as a 60-year-old high-income male (Case & Deaton, 2005). This is partly explained by health behavior. Higher SES people are less likely to smoke, to drink heavily, or to be obese (Marmot, 2006).

The higher prevalence of unhealthy behaviors in lower socioeconomic classes is seen to be one of the mechanisms linking lower SES to poor health. The contribution of unhealthy behaviors, such as smoking, alcohol consumption, and poor diet, are shown to explain 12% to 72%

---

[5]Thus, health care providers may consider alternative motivating strategies to stressing the health benefits accruing 10, 15, or 20 years in the future. For example, strategies that emphasize more proximate benefits should be considered for the least future-oriented patients.

of the socioeconomic differences in mortality (Stringhini et al., 2010). Moreover, evidence suggests that these behaviors are traceable to early childhood experience (Cutler et al., 2010). Public health interventions that improve individual health behaviors have the potential to increase the population's health, as well as reduce inequities in health.

The associations between SES and health are graded, such that with every decrease in SES, there is increasing risk. What matters is the relative income, not the absolute income level. Within developed nations, there is little relationship between per capita income and life expectancy. In 2003, for example, in Greece, the life expectancy (78.3) was 1.9 years longer than in the United States (77.4), in spite of the U.S. having twice the income of Greece ($37,562 vs. $19,954) (Marmot, 2006). Thus, absolute income is not a very good guide to longevity. Even relatively affluent groups exhibit worse health than their higher SES counterparts. Thus, income inequality, or relative position, is a better indicator as a social determinant of health. In this framework, a person's income matters only insofar as it distinguishes him from his neighbor. The SES factors do not work individually but are likely to accumulate in low SES environments.

Education

The health production model assumes that educated individuals are more efficient producers of health (i.e., can produce the same amount of health with fewer inputs, or can produce more health with the same inputs) than those with less education. Thus, educated people experience a higher rate of return to a given stock of health. More educated individuals in the United States report better health and face lower mortality risk. Evidence shows that in the 1980s and 1990s, virtually all gains in life expectancy occurred among highly educated groups (Marmot, 2006). For example, in 2000, the difference between poor black men and affluent White women was more than 14 years (66.9 years vs. 81.1 years). Analysis of compulsory schooling laws in the early twentieth century showed that individuals born in states that forced them to remain in school longer enjoyed significantly higher survival rates in adulthood (Cutler et al., 2010). Another study reports that since unemployment rates lower the opportunity cost of staying in school, teenagers facing unemployment attain higher levels of education and are healthier adults (Arkes, 2001). Thus, education contributes to the growing disparities in life expectancy for richer and poorer Americans. When policymakers debate the merits of increasing access to education, they rarely consider improvements in the health of the population.

Those with more years of schooling tend to have better health and healthier lifestyle (Marmot, 2006). Better-educated parents (especially mothers) have healthier children. For example, for women in the United States, a minimum of 2 years of college decreases the likelihood of smoking during pregnancy by 5.8% points (Currie & Moretti, 2003). Those with more education are less likely to smoke, drink excessively, carry excess weight, or use illegal drugs. The better educated also obtain more preventive care (e.g., flu shots and mammograms), manage existing conditions more effectively (e.g., diabetes and hypertension), and makes more use of safety devices such as seat belts and smoke detectors.

It is shown that individuals from lower SES are more resistant to changing their unhealthy behaviors compared with higher SES counterparts (Cutler et al., 2010). For example, much of the long-term decline in smoking has taken place in the higher SES groups, with the result that smoking is increasingly concentrated in poorer and socially disadvantaged groups. In 1965, the year following the first Surgeon General's report, less than 3% points separated the prevalence of smoking among college graduates (33.7%) from that of Americans who did not graduate from high school (36.5%). By 1997, prevalence among college graduates had fallen by nearly two-thirds, to 11.6%. Among people without a high school diploma, in contrast, prevalence had fallen by only one-sixth (to 30.4%). The gap had grown to almost 19 points.

There is also a possibility of reverse relationship between health and education. The expectation of a longer and healthier life may motivate more investment in human capital. The affluent, well-educated population finds the future, especially the prospect of retirement, far more attractive than the lower-income population for whom the future indicates only continuing economic worries (Fuchs, 1986). As a consequence, members of low SES groups may heavily discount[6] the future promised by not smoking.

Good health allows children to attain more schooling and also makes them more likely to become healthy adults. Case et al. (2005) show that in Britain, adolescents who were born with low birthweight or suffered from illness in childhood have worse schooling outcomes. In a study of the long-run effects of the 1918 flu epidemic in the United States, Almond (2006) shows that children exposed to the epidemic *in utero* had lower educational attainment as adults.

---

[6]The person's discount rate refers to the weight an individual places on future happiness relative to current happiness. The extent to which an individual is forward-looking, or the rate at which one discount future happiness, varies across people and can determine optimal health stock.

Cognitive ability represents a significant part of the link between education and health (Cutler et al., 2010). Education affects cognition, which in turn affects the ability to process information regarding healthy behaviors. Individuals with higher levels of education tend to have better understanding of their symptoms and have better communication skills to explain these to health providers than individuals with lower levels of education. Another mechanism through which educational attainment may affect health capital accumulation is discounting that leads to the positive correlation between education and health observed empirically. Fuch (1986) shows that one possible reason for high correlation between individual's health status and the length of schooling is that attending to one's health and attending school are both aspects of investment in human capital. Thus, the same person who has accumulated a great deal of human capital in the form of schooling may, for the same reason, have made substantial investments in health (or have them made for him).

Income

There is a gradient or stepwise relationship between income and health. Being poor is bad for individual health and bodyweight (Sobal & Stunkard, 1989). Income and wealth improve access to health inputs such as medical care and food, and health improves one's ability to participate in labor market and earn income.

Adult health also has a large effect on adult income. Among adults, the negative impact of poor health on income and wealth is attributable to a decline in wage earnings. Smith (1999) finds that the onset of a new illness reduces household wealth even among households with health insurance. Negative health stocks strongly predict retirement and reduced labor force participation (Smith, 1999). Parental income has strong protective effects on children's health. The parental economic resources protect children's health and their potential economic success later in life. As children age, the accumulation of health inputs continue into adulthood. Thus, healthier children become wealthier healthier adults, as they attain more schooling.

Rank

The relationships of education and income variables with health are based on economic approach. These variables operate through individuals' preferences and their capacities to purchase health inputs, process information, and participate in economic life. Low SES (including education and income) produces psychosocial stress due to feelings of subordination and lack of control. Individuals with higher income and education enjoy better health because of the individuals' position in a social hierarchy, and position in the hierarchy shows a strong correlation with mortality risk. Marmot (2006) explains that status is partly related to how we see ourselves and how others see us, but it is also related to our social circumstances, or how a particular community intensifies or buffers differences in social position. According to Marmot, status is more important than genetics, access to health care, and health behavior such as eating and smoking. Our position in the hierarchy very much relates to how much control we have over our life and our opportunities for full social engagement.

Data from the Whitehall study of British Civil Servants[7] (Marmot, 2006) showed that people at each employment grade in government service experienced worse health and had higher mortality than those in the grade immediately above them. The study demonstrates that there is a significant relationship between mortality and grade of employment. These mortality differences have behavioral precursors; higher ranking officials display a lower obesity rate, a lower propensity to smoke, and higher propensities to exercise and eat fruits and vegetables. Employment grade also associates positively with a sense of control over one's health and one's work, job satisfaction, social support, and the absence of stressful life events. Given that most subjects of these studies enjoy a high degree of job security and have access to adequate earnings, common interpretations of their results place more weight on psychosocial factors than on material considerations.

Wilkinson (1996) presents the idea that subordination worsens health more than domination improves it, leading to the prediction that inequalities in income and wealth are detrimental to population health. The relative income deprivation affects health by insulting humans' innate sense of fairness. The effects of such deprivation are likely to accumulate over the course of a lifetime. Thus, countries with more income inequality—and therefore more poor people—would experience worse population health outcomes. In this framework, an extra dollar given to

---

[7]The British Whitehall II cohort was established in 1985 to examine the socioeconomic gradient in health and disease among 10,308 civil servants. They were aged 35–55 years and working in 20 departments in London, England. Their position consists of three levels: high (administrative), intermediate (professional or executive), and low (clerical or support) grades. Administrative grades in the British civil services represent the highest grade. The participants are White workers with universal access to health care. This sample may not be representative of the general population in terms of socioeconomic spectrum, but this may also mean that socioeconomic differences in the general population are even larger.

a poor person influences his health far more than the same dollar would affect a rich person's health.[8]

The key mechanism in the link between rank and health is the fight-or-flight response, a chain of biochemical and physiological reactions to threats that occurs in most animals and humans. The physiological reactions involve heightened heart rate and a redistribution of blood away from essential organs toward the skeletal muscles to prepare the animal to protect itself against immediate danger. However, repeated exposure to the biochemical events associated with fight-or-flight takes its toll on the body, resulting in what is known as *"allostatic load"* among humans. Increases in allostatic load[9] raise mortality risk and cardiovascular disease (CVD) risk, hasten cognitive and physical decline, and suppress the immune system (McEwen, 1998). Chronic exposure to stress, and inadequate stress buffering, is also associated with the shortening of special clusters of DNA at the ends of chromosomes, called telomeres (considered a biological clock). Shortening or telomere is thought to be an integral part of the aging process. Thus, prolonged stress accelerates aging and impairs immunity system.[10]

The workplace is a context that provides almost routine exposure to chronic psychosocial stressors. Work related stress may include factors such as the demands of the job, the ability to have control over decisions, and the degree of social support within the workplace. The lower you are in the hierarchy, the lower the level of control you have over your work. People who have more control over their work have better health. People with low job control have about twice the incidence of coronary heart disease, as compared with those with high control (Marmot, 2006).

The gap between demand and control[11] (or *job strain*) is the main occupational stress. Job strain can be considered as a type of chronic stress.

---

[8]However, some studies have challenged the association between income inequality and health. Their findings show that changes in income inequality explain little, if any, of the mortality rates.

[9]The allostatic load (the impact of lifelong experiences of "wear and tear") refers to the continued and unproductive activation of the stress response, including the failure to shut-off this response when it is not needed.

[10]Sapolsky's research on baboons (2004) finds that subordinate males display higher levels of glucocortoids, hormones that are secreted in response to stress. The subordinates also perform poorly on a range of health measures, including blood pressure, cholesterol levels, and body fatness. When researchers induce changes in baboons' social standing, the same patterns occur, implying that this is not merely the result of genetic sorting.

[11]Jobs with high demands require an excessive amount of work output, usually under a variety of constraints (i.e., time pressure, performance expectations, and layoff possibilities). Those in jobs with low decision latitude have little control over their assigned tasks, work that is often characterized by its simplicity and repetitive nature.

The accumulated evidence supports an association between job strain and CVD incidence and mortality. Job strain is also closely related to SES, since individuals with lower SES are more likely to hold jobs that are higher in demands and, particularly, lower in control. High BMI has also been observed among those high job demands and low levels of decision latitude (Dallman, 2010).

Gallo, Bogart, Vranceanu, and Matthews (2005) developed *the reserve capacity model* as a framework for understanding how emotional factors in particular might contribute to SES disparities in health. The reserve capacity is conceptualized as an aggregate "bank" of interpersonal (e.g., social support and social integration) and intrapersonal resources (e.g., perceived control, self-efficacy, optimism, and self-esteem). These resources can dampen physiological stress responses that foster disease vulnerability, or they can help attenuate stress perceptions, facilitate positive outcomes, and promote adaptive coping. Individuals with lower SES tend to report greater depression, anxiety, and hostility-emotional factors that subsequently relate to health risk factors and outcomes (Marmot, 2006). Low resources and stress also relate to unhealthy behaviors, such as smoking, poor nutrition, and reduced sleep.

For example, in a small study of Hispanic women (Gallo et al., 2005), psychological resources (aggregated optimism, mastery, self-esteem, and social support) accounted for one-third of the relationship between SES and abdominal obesity, which is a risk factor for elevated risk of CVD and Type 2 diabetes. The study demonstrates that a deficit in resilient resources may link SES with risk for the metabolic syndrome, most likely via physiological stress responses and health behaviors, as indicated below:

Low SES $\rightarrow$ Reserve Capacity $\rightarrow$ Health Risk

In sum, psychosocial factors such as stress, negative emotions, and social isolation relate to major health outcomes, including CVD and all cause mortality. In addition, these factors vary by SES so that individuals with low SES show relatively high levels of psychosocial risk. Psychosocial resources relate directly to physical and mental health. Moreover, social status can shape appraisals in a way that further increases stress burden. For example, research suggests that individuals with low SES and those previously exposed to racial discrimination formulate negative interpretations of even ambiguous social interactions, and that individuals with low SES view their social worlds as hostile and unfriendly relative to those with higher SES. Over time, the wear and tear from repeated physiological stress responses, combined with unhealthy behavioral coping strategies, take their toll, increasing vulnerability to disease.

THE LIFE COURSE PERSPECTIVE

Circumstances in early life play a crucial role in determining the association between SES and health throughout adulthood. A person's past social experiences become written into the physiology and psychology of their body. Accumulation of individual life experiences shape the course of people's later years. From a life course perspective, the socioeconomic disparity in health and disease results from the processes of accumulation of advantage or disadvantage. In other words, disadvantaged youths are more likely than their counterparts to become disadvantaged adults. For example, poor health during childhood is associated with reduced educational attainment, lower social status, and more health problem in adulthood, suggesting health is an important mechanism through which economic status is transmitted (Cutler et al., 2010). Poor children suffer more insults to their health than richer ones (Currie, Vigna, Moretti, & Pathania, 2009). For example, poor children are more likely to have many chronic conditions, such as asthma and ADHD (32.4% of poor children vs. 26.5% other children). This disparity between rich and poor children rises with age.

Moreover, the poor are at higher risk for obesity than the rich. Hence, the growth in obesity will exacerbate existing differences in health between rich and poor since many diseases, such as heart disease and diabetes, are related to obesity. Research shows that overweight adolescents are likely to attain lower education than normal weight children and adolescents. Two reasons for this are that obese students are exposed to stigma and psychological pressure and have a higher number of sick days (Datar & Sturm, 2006). Since learning begets learning, this education gap is likely to widen during adult life, with important effects on productivity.

The research evidence shows that persistent poverty is likely to have worse effects on health than transitory poverty. Since health is a stock that will be affected by past investments, children with low health may be less able to utilize new investments in their health capital for production of a wide range of future capacities. Thus, low SES in childhood is related to poorer future adult health, even in adults who are no longer of lower SES (Heckman, 2007).

The fetal origins literature strongly suggests that conditions in utero affect not only birth weight but features such as basic metabolism, which in turn affect future health outcomes. The work of David Barker, known as the "Barker hypothesis," is that events in the womb have long-lasting effects on health throughout life, and perhaps particularly for health outcomes that express themselves in late life (Barker, Eriksson, Forsen, & Osmond, 2002). This is also known as *biological programming*, which refers to marginally incomplete fetal development, of which low birthweight is a nonspecific marker. The associations between low birthweight and later disease have been shown to be independent of influences such as SES and cigarette smoking. Barker maintains that fetuses starved in utero may develop more efficient metabolisms, which then place them at higher risk for future obesity, heart disease, and diabetes. Malnutrition retards brain and nerve formation, which leads to learning disabilities and higher rates of schizophrenia; it disrupts hormone production, which interferes with the development of vital organs such as the gut, heart, and lungs, making them weaker and more prone to later failure. Some of the damage is reversible if proper nutrition is restored. Fogel argues that malnourished humans wear out more quickly and are less efficient at every age. In short, hunger effectively destroys the mental, social, and productive capacities of entire population.

Severe nutritional deprivation in utero or in early childhood can cause permanent cognitive impairments. For example, consider the "Dutch Hunger Winter" of November 1944 to April 1945, when Dutch citizens were reduced to starvation by the Nazi occupation. Adults in utero during the time of the famine were more likely than those in the surrounding cohorts to suffer various health impairments, including disorders of the central nervous system, heart disease, and antisocial personality disorders (Doblhammer, 2004).

In child development research, self-regulation is important in the capacity for stress management and governing health behavior. Self-regulation refers to deliberative processes that enable an individual to guide his/her thoughts or affect behavior or attention. Children with low SES are more likely to have deficit in self-regulation, suggesting that experiences of the stress of low SES and unhealthy behaviors have common roots early life and should be considered part of the same adult pathway. Emotional dysregulation and insecurity in childhood may lead to mistrust of others, poor social and coping skills, and feelings of depression, anxiety, and anger.

In sum, there is a strong evidence of correlation between socioeconomic measures of parental background and child health. Children of poor or less educated parents are in worse health, on average than other children. The literature indicates that adversity is not randomly distributed; instead it tends to accumulate on top of previous disadvantage. Consequently, any single misfortune tends to affect the most vulnerable individuals who have accumulated the greatest number of previous handicaps. The policy implication is to provide good nutrition, health and preventive care services, and adequate social and economic resources, before first pregnancies, during pregnancy, and in infancy, to improve growth and development before birth and throughout infancy, and reduce the risk of disease and malnutrition in infancy. Research shows that prenatal participation in the U.S. WIC (Supplemental Nutrition for Women, Infants, and Children) program is associated with higher test scores (Smith, 2009). WIC is a program that provides coupons redeemable for specific foods to women, infants, and children deemed to be "nutritionally at risk" (David Rush et al., 1988). Thus, better nutrition could improve cognitive performance.

DISPARITY IN OBESITY

Adult body weight and obesity are negatively related to social and economic advantages. Obesity is more prevalent among the lower socioeconomic groups, especially among women. For example, Chou, Grossman, and Saffer (2004) find that years of formal schooling completed and real household income have negative effects on BMI and the probability of being obese for U.S. adults.

Several studies have shown a stronger inverse SES gradient among women than among men in economically developed countries. Women of lower income are approximately 50% more likely to be obese than those with higher income levels. One reason for this is a strong norm among higher SES women to be slim.[12] In the western societies, thinness has become a status symbol, whereas obesity is often considered as a sign of laziness and lack of self-control (Oliver & Lee, 2005). It is possible that persons of high status may internalize the symbolic value of a thin and a healthy lifestyle (in line with their class) and at the same time face exposure to workplace environment that likewise promote these values. Women in higher social classes may be more susceptible to media messages and/or better able to pursue methods of achieving the ideal body weight. However, the link between SES and obesity in the United States has weakened. The disparity in obesity rates has declined over the past three decades. The relative difference in the prevalence of obesity between low- and high-SES groups decreased from 50% in 1970–1974 to 14% in 1999–2000. Our obesogenic environment may make it increasingly difficult for women of any class to maintain resistance.

Studies reveal that parental education is inversely associated with adiposity than any other SES indicators (occupation or income). Parental education compared with other SES indicators is more protective against obesity. Furthermore, since obesity develops over a lengthy period, so bodyweight may reflect an accumulation of the effects of SES.

---

[12]Another reason is that women constitute the majority of adults receiving public aid from government. There is some evidence that public assistance programs cause recipients to overeat and gain weight (Smith, 2009).

For example, low SES may raise weight by influencing patterns of eating habits and physical activity later in life. Similarly, Powell (2009) shows that youth in the higher SES families are significantly less likely to be overweight compared with their low-SES counterparts. For example, 7.5% of youths from high-income families are overweight compared with 11.8% and 14.8% from middle- and low-income families, respectively (Hu, 2008).

In non Western and developing countries, there is a positive association between socioeconomic position (SEP) and obesity. Being poor in the poorest nations (per capita less than $800 per year) of the world is associated with being underweight and malnourished, whereas the poor in more affluent countries have an increased obesity risk. However, as the Western lifestyle (decreasing physical activity and increased consumption of high energy-dense foods) become more prevalent, obesity can be expected to rise. For example, the rapid modernization of China has produced an alarming spike in the rate of obesity and diabetes among their populations. Western diet, high in fat and sugar, puts them in danger of developing Type 2 diabetes. At the same time, large shifts towards less physically demanding work have been observed worldwide. Thus, unlike previous centuries, increased weight is not a sign of improved health, the rapid increase in body weight indicate growing share of population is becoming obese. In sum, the economic growth, modernization, nutritional change, and globalization of food markets, have reduced the differences in obesity rates between developing and developed countries.

AVAILABILITY OF HEALTHY FOOD

Lack of availability and high costs of food are two constraints to eating more healthfully. Neighborhood characteristics influence obesity and health. The literature suggests that living in poor neighborhoods in the United States generally means having less access to healthy foods and greater exposure to high-calorie foods (Drewnowski & Darmon, 2005). There are fewer places to buy healthy foods, as well as fewer supermarkets per capita. Low SES households are closer to small convenience stores that tend to stock fewer fresh fruits and vegetables, and offer ready-made, packaged products with high calories and fat. Individuals with low SES also live in places saturated by fast-food restaurants and liquor stores. For example, Chicago neighborhoods close to fast-food outlets and far from grocery stores have higher average BMI (Gallagher, 2006).

People living in poorer areas face somewhat higher grocery prices and have less physical access to healthy foods and greater access to fast foods. Living in a neighborhood with access to multiple full-service supermarkets, plentiful safe options for physical activity, and options for walking for transportation may decease one's likelihood for becoming obese. It is also possible that the consumption of healthy products affects their supply. Over time, low demand for fruits and vegetables is likely to decrease their availability in local stores.

POVERTY AND OBESITY

Economic factors may help explain why low-income individuals are least likely to eat healthy diets. Low-income families spend a higher proportion of their budget on food relative to their affluent counterparts. Thus, they have less discretionary income to buy expensive healthy food. According to economic logic, consuming energy-dense foods (e.g., doughnuts, potato chips) and energy-dense diets, are important strategies used by low-income consumers to stretch the food budget. Energy-dense foods carry a lower price tag, which allows for a higher energy consumption at a lower cost. For example, cookies and potato chips provide 1,200 calories per dollar, whereas fresh carrots provide 250 calories per dollar. Thus, the observed SES gradient in diet quality may be mediated by food prices. Low-cost foods are more affordable and more accessible for low-income families. A consumer survey found that those making less than $10,000 were the highest purchasers of processed snack cakes, whereas those making more than $250,000 bought the least (Darmon & Drewnowski, 2008). The food they eat turns into habit: it becomes part of their personal culture. Darmon and Drewnowski (2008) argue that the promotion of high-cost healthier diets to low-income people is not likely to be successful without considering food cost. These promotion policies assume that all foods cost the same, and consumers' choice will be improved by increasing awareness and motivation without considerations of the diet costs. They demonstrate that obesity in America is mostly an economic issue. That is the rising obesity rates reflect the increasingly unequal distributions of incomes and wealth.

Moreover, palatable energy-dense foods have been associated with diminished satiation and satiety, may be the principal reasons for overeating and weight gain. In contrast, bulky foods with a high water content are said to promote a feeling of fullness, which leads to reduced energy intakes. Foods that are energy-dense provide more sensory enjoyment and more pleasure than do foods that are not. Therefore, the burden of obesity and diabetes in rich societies falls disproportionately on the poor. Thus, obesity is becoming a disease of the poor.

SOCIAL NORMS AND NETWORKS

The study of social networks[13] provides a unique insight to our health choices. The spread of obesity in social networks appears to be another factor in the obesity epidemic. Like any other phenomenon, obesity can spread within social networks. People are connected, and so is their health. Weight spreads through a variety of social ties from person to person. Spouses and siblings influence each other. Coworkers influence each other, too. Recent work in the U.S. suggests that social networks appear to be important in "transmitting" obesity (Christakis & Fowler, 2007). The study argues that the "fault" for the behavior of excess does not lie in the individual; rather it is the fault of the wider society and the context in which individuals finds themselves.

How do social networks affect someone's weight? People are connected in vast social networks. Our connections affect every aspect of our daily lives. Our behaviors such as food intakes or smoking are influenced by people we have never met. For example, students with studious roommates become more studious (Christakis & Fowler, 2009). Diners sitting next to heavy eaters eat more food (Wansink, 2006). But how is obesity contagious? There are two mechanisms: behavioral imitation and norms.

What spreads from person to person is what social scientists call a *norm*, which is a shared expectation about what is appropriate. A social norm creates shared expectations about how a group of people (reference group) ought to behave.[14] For example, we might look at those around us and see that they are gaining weight, and this might change our ideas about acceptable body size. When many people start gaining weight, it can reset our expectations about what it actually means to be overweight. For example, in the U.S., obesity rates are much higher among lower income groups. The real epidemic, the one at the root of obesity, is an

---

[13]A social network, like a group, is a collection of people. They allow groups to do things that individuals alone cannot. The whole is greater than the sum of its part. For example, having extra friends may create all kinds of benefits for your health, even if this other person does not actually do anything in particular for you. The simplest social network is a pair of people, a dyad, such as husband and wife. In general, social networks evolve organically from the natural tendency of each person to seek out and make many friends, such as a single dormitory in a college, or an entire community, or the worldwide network that links us all.

[14]As Elster (1989) notes, social norms are sustained by the feelings of shame and guilt. If you deviate from the prescribed body shape too much, you will feel badly about yourself. In other words, it makes you less unhappy to be obese if others around you are obese. Thus, body dissatisfaction can be the result of the discrepancy between perceived and ideal body sizes. This also suggests that people's decisions with respect to their food consumption or their exercise may be due less to their absolute weight than their "relative" weight: that is, their weight as compared with that of the people around them.

epidemic of attitudes. Overweight is not the problem; it is a symptom of the problem.[15]

From an economic perspective, a person's weight preference may depend on relative weight (your BMI divided by the average BMI in your peer). In other words, people have a utility function defined on relative weight and rationally choose a weight after observing the weights of their peers (Blanchflower, Oswald, & van Landeghem, 2009). For a variety of reasons, it may be easier to be fat in a society that is fat. In a world of comparisons, people will often emulate each other in a kind of keeping-up-with-the-Joneses sense, and fatness can then in principle spread in a way that would have the appearance of a contagious effect. For example, for a given level of BMI, highly educated people are the most likely to see themselves as fat. This suggests that people have different comparison groups. The highly educated hold themselves to a thinner standard.

Imitation is another way obesity might spread from person to person. If you start eating fattening foods, your friends might follow suit. Behavior imitations can be either conscious or unconscious. When we see someone eat, our mirror neurons fire in the same part of the brain that would be activated if we ourselves were eating. It is as if our brains practice doing something that we have merely been watching. And this practice in turn makes it easier for us to exhibit the same behavior in the future.

The spread of obesity in a large social network highlight the necessity of approaching obesity as a public health problem. Group-level interventions may be more successful and also more cost-effective. The approach can also be exploited to spread positive health behaviors, in part because people's perceptions of their own risk of illness may depend on the people around them. Weight loss programs that modify the person's social network (provide peer support) tend to be more successful. In fact, programs such as Alcohol Anonymous or weight loss groups are explicitly designed to create a set of artificial social network ties. Evidence on smoking behavior shows that for every 10 people who stop smoking, there will be another two who in the long run do not smoke as a consequence, an indirect effect of 20% (Rosen, 1989). Trends toward a decline in smoking around the world have surely been reinforced by social diffusion.

In short, health behaviors like staying healthy or smoking pass from friend to friend almost as if they were contagious viruses. Staying healthy is not just a matter of your genes and your diet, it is also a product, in

---

[15]Social norm may amplify the effect of price declines on the BMI distribution. For example, a fall in price will have a positive direct effect on caloric intake, which will move the BMI distribution to the right. The shift in BMI will be amplified through an increase in social norms as the cost of overeating will fall. For example, Chen and Meltzer (2008) argue that Chinese obesity is increasing because of changing norms and social contagion. From the health policy perspective, social norms will magnify the effect of prevention policies.

part, of your sheer proximity to other healthy people. The powerful effects of social networks on individual behaviors suggest that people do not have complete control over their choices. Our connections to others affect our capacity for free fill. This suggests that a more effective approach to understanding obesity is to focus on the structure of a person's social network, namely their structural position rather than their SEP.

CONCLUSION

The social determinants perspective on obesity requires attention to "the causes of the causes." This means moving beyond the individual to explore potential determinants occurring at multiple levels. These factors include SEP, psychosocial characteristics, and social environment. For example, chronic exposure to psychosocial stress may increase the likelihood of "comfort eating." Poor health may restrict a family's capacity to earn income or to accumulate assets by limiting work or by raising medical expenses. Education continues to be a powerful determinant of health, but to a great extent because of its impact on behaviors rather than its association with resources. In childhood, parental resources (education and income) have a potent effect on health. Insults to child health may persist into adulthood, constraining adults in the labor market. From the health policy perspective, obesity prevention needs to pay attention to social determinants of health to address inequalities in health, such as socioeconomic variables, income inequalities, and social inequities.

6

Decision Making Over Time

INTRODUCTION

An important concept in behavioral economics is to examine how people make decisions over time. When confronted with a choice of whether to overeat, individuals can opt for one of two outcomes: an immediate benefit of pleasure or a delayed benefit (or uncertain benefit), such as health. In economic jargon, these are known as *intertemporal decisions*. These decisions have a time dimension, meaning that they involve trade-offs between costs and benefits occurring at different times. Such choices pervade our lives, from daily decisions to ones that can have lifelong consequences (e.g., dietary choices, savings, education, and marriage).

Health behavior decisions, such as eating habits, exercise, smoking, getting periodic checkups, and so forth, have consequences that are typically realized only after a long period of time. It has been estimated that as much as 40% of all premature mortality in the United States is the result of unhealthy behavior (McGinnis, 1999), which represents decisions favoring immediate benefits at the expense of delayed costs. Achieving and maintaining health typically involve incurring a current cost in exchange for the chance of some future benefit. For example, weight loss involves foregoing immediate pleasure to gain future health benefits. Lying in the sun provides an attractive tan in the near future but may lead to adverse health consequences in the distant future, such as unattractive wrinkles or a greater risk of skin cancer.

The concept of choice over time provides a conceptual framework in explaining the human taste for instant gratification (and excess consumption) and provides principles to guide behavior. It explains key decision-making biases that ordinarily lead to self-harming behavior and shows how they can be used to promote healthy behaviors. The main goal is to introduce the concept of time preference and its determinants, and time-inconsistent preferences for immediate gratification. *Time inconsistent preferences* mean that people have a present-biased preference. We often want gratification right now, such as when eating highly caloric foods while planning a diet starting tomorrow.

TIME PREFERENCE AND DISCOUNTING

Time preference (or *discount rate*) is an economic concept that refers to the rate at which people discount the future relative to the present. It represents an individual's willingness to give up current consumption in exchange for future consumption. Time preference is a measure of an individual's overall tendency to prefer smaller, sooner rewards to larger later ones. *Positive time preference* motivates a person to act myopically (present oriented). A person with positive time preference requires more than one unit of future consumption to compensate for the loss of a unit of current consumption. In general, individuals with high rates of positive time preference will tend to invest less in future-oriented activities, such as health and education.

A given level of time preference can correspond to a higher or lower discount rate. The *discount rate* refers to the weight an individual places on future outcomes relative to current outcomes. *Discounting of delayed rewards* refers to the observation that the value of a delayed reward is reduced (or considered to be worth less) when compared with the value of an immediate reward. Higher discount rates give greater weight to benefits and costs accruing sooner than do lower discount rates. For example, a high discount rate may reduce a person's willingness to forgo current caloric intake for the future benefit of lower weight. Farmers with high discount rates are more likely to plant crops with a short harvesting time and a low yield than crops with a longer harvesting time but a higher yield.

Reasons for Discounting

How can delay reduce value? In general, two factors explain discounting. The first is the opportunity costs of delay. The interest lost from delaying the receipt of money or paying it out too soon is one example of an opportunity cost. For example, if the interest rate is 5%, waiting 1 year for $105 instead of taking $100 immediately would cost the decision maker $5 in interest.

The second basis is pure time preference (impatience) or the desire to avoid delay of consumption, meaning that a given amount of utility (happiness) is preferred the earlier it arrives. This is the psychological discomfort associated with self-denial. Thus individuals are willing to accept a small sum of money today in exchange for a larger sum in the future. For example, many individuals are willing to buy cheaper cars with less fuel efficiency instead of a more expensive car that will incur lower fuel costs over its lifetime.

In general, the preference for an immediate or a distant outcome is a function of the value of the respective outcomes and their delays, that is, the time until they can be realized. For example, a given reward delivered after a long delay is less attractive than the same reward delivered after a short delay. So, getting $1,000 tomorrow is preferred to $2,000 2 years from now. Similarly, losing $1,000 tomorrow hurts more than losing $2,000 2 years from now. This explains why people have an easier time spending money on credit cards as opposed to spending real money. In general, the delay until the arrival of higher outcome is seen as a cost and is weighed against the distant benefits.

A Normative Basis of Discounting

Choice over time has an uncontroversial normative principle.[1] A long time ago philosophers argued that pure time discounting may be undesirable—in other words, that one time is as good as another and it is immoral to discount (Frank, 2003). They viewed equal treatment of present and future as a norm of behavior. To attach less weight to a future benefit merely because it arrives in the future is as irrational as preferring a benefit on Mondays over Tuesdays. They noted that impatience for future rewards usually made people poorer in the long run. A person who discounts the future very heavily will ruin his health, his family life, and his finances for the sake of short-term pleasures. In short, these philosophers recognized the discounting of delayed outcomes as an important barrier to humans' ability to maximize their resources. For example, a person who ignores the long-term impact of smoking and high-fat food will likely have a shorter life expectancy.

These philosophers, however, recognized that the tendency to discount future rewards is due to our "defective telescopic faculty." Just as distant objects appear to be smaller than those close up, so do temporally remote rewards appear to be smaller than present ones. In other words, discounting behavior is similar to an optical illusion than to a motivational bias (Elster, 2006). It is a widely accepted principle that the intensity of sensual experiences declines with distance (the Weber–Fechner rule). The same limitation applies to our capacity to contemplate the future; consequently we place less value on future benefit and cost.[2]

---

[1]A normative statement expresses a judgment and addresses what should be rather than what is. In contrast, positive economics deals with description and explanations of economic relationships.

[2]Similarly, the decay of past experience means that it is difficult to learn from experience.

FACTORS AFFECTING DISCOUNTING

What determines the level of time preference? Why do humans differ in the extent to which they discount delayed rewards? The following sections briefly discuss determinants of time preference. These factors explain why people care less about a future consequence.

Uncertainty

People tend to equate temporal distance with uncertainty; that is, the distant future is riskier than the near future. This means a proximal reward may be preferred over a distant reward in the same way as a likely reward is preferred over an unlikely reward. For instance, a lifetime of learning not to trust others to deliver what they promise in the future may play a role in delay-discounting rates. Individuals who grow up in an untrusted environment will have the tendency to grab whatever is immediately available. Similarly, the short duration and uncertainty of life influence time preference. This may explain why, for example, there is an inverse relationship between saving rates (a proxy for time perspective) in different countries and fear of nuclear war. Poor health is an indicator of mortality and will therefore increase one's uncertainty about whether future reward will be received.

An evolutionary perspective provides an explanation for the link between uncertainty and discounting. Throughout evolutionary history, future rewards have been uncertain (Logue, 1988). Our instinct is to seize the reward at hand, and resisting this instinct is hard. In prehistoric human environments, the availability of food was uncertain. Because of the variability of the environment, the prospect of waiting for a delayed reward was risky. Like other animals, humans would survive and reproduce if they had a strong tendency to grab the smaller, immediate reward and forgo the larger but delayed reward. If you were out hunting for turkeys to eat, a bird in the hand would be worth two (or more than two) in the bush.[3] Evolution therefore has given people and other animals[4]

---

[3]It was unlikely that a man would become unhealthy if he gorged himself when food was available. Rather, gorging himself would serve to effectively bridge the frequent periods when food was scarce.

[4]For example, consider the choice of a mate. Widow birds prefer males with long tails (a sign of male quality). So a female confronted with a short-tailed male faces a dilemma: settle for the short-tailed male or keep looking. Viewed from the lens of evolutionary approach, the appropriate behavior is a fit between decision mechanisms and the environment in which the animal operates. Thus, living in a competitive environment (high uncertainty), waiting imposes opportunity costs for birds with short life spans. Thus, uncertainty motivates the bird to settle for a less than ideal mate.

a strong desire for immediate rewards and even stronger tendency to avoid immediate pain. At the same time, counter to our tendency for immediate consumption, human reason has evolved an ability to predict the future, and human society has evolved to reduce the uncertainty of distant rewards. However, the existence of the capacity for perceiving long-term consequences does not imply that it will be used. In addition to cognitive capacity, people need to be motivated to take those consequences into account.

Age

Why do young people sometimes behave as if there is no tomorrow? Young people are more likely than older ones to seek new experiences and discount future consequences. As infants, we all dwell in the land of immediate gratification and self-interest, but over time, and under appropriate parental influences, we learn not to grab toys away from our playmates, hit our siblings, or eat an entire box of cookies 20 minutes before our dinner.

A study by Green, Fry, and Myerson (1994) compared the discounting of hypothetical monetary rewards among children (mean age of 12.1 years), young adults (mean age of 20.3 years), and older adults (mean age of 67.9 years). The results showed that children discounted the most, older adults discounted the least, and the young adults' discounting was intermediate between them. The finding shows a U-shape between age and discounting. That is, discounting decreases through young adulthood and middle age and then increases again beyond retirement age.

Childhood and adolescence, in particular, are points of the life cycle that may be associated with greater uncertainty and perhaps this is an important factor contributing to the widely held view that the young live as if tomorrow will never come. As we age, we tend to experience more certainty and therefore may consider the future more. Thus, as a person gets older and wiser, his or her apparent discount curve gets smaller.[5] Research has shown that experience of life events that bear lessons about time can change one's time preferences (Liu & Aaker, 2008). For instance, the experience with death of someone close induces young adults to reflect upon their long-term futures and become more long-term focused. Having a vivid view of the future ahead is a sign of social maturity for young adults.

---

[5]Mark Twain once said that "life would be infinitely happier if we could only be born at the age of eighty and gradually approach eighteen." The movie *The Curious Case of Benjamin Button* (2008) is a dramatic illustration of the idea of aging backward.

Developmental Course of Discounting

Resisting short-term rewards in favor of longer-term rewards requires a capacity to envision the distant future. For youths this ability is "under construction." In adolescents, the emotional (motivational) brain areas are particularly active, whereas the part of the brain that is supposed to inhibit impulses is not fully developed (Goldberg, 2009). Thus, impulsive decision making in adolescents may be related to a relatively underdeveloped cognitive brain (orbitofrontal cortex) combined with overactive emotional brain (limbic reward system).[6] The developmental course may explain why teenagers often seem so excessively self-centered, and why they may fail to think about the effects of their behaviors.[7] This also implies that many of the future consequences of an unhealthy behavior (such as drug abuse, for example) will be more heavily discounted by youths than by adults. There is now widespread agreement that impulsivity plays a key role in the initiation and development of drug use problems (Bickel et al., 2007).

Impulsivity

Many psychologists believe that impulsivity (a persistent tendency to behave in an impulsive manner) is a trait. The trait of impulsivity refers to a chronic and general tendency to act on impulses. People with an impulsive personality are simply more prone to be in an impulsive mood and they tend show intolerance to delay of gratification or delay aversion (Madden & Bickel, 2010). Impulsivity[8] makes it more difficult for some individuals to resist the psychological discomfort associated with self-denial.[9] So, individuals with impulsive traits will be at greater risk for numerous problems, such as substance abuse.

---

[6]Children with attention-deficit hyperactivity disorder experience the greatest delays in brain maturation in those areas of the cortex most involved in attention and motor control. Many youth eventually seem to grow out of the disorder.

[7]Consider the news about the 14-times Olympic gold medal winner Michael Phelps who was caught with cannabis pipe (01/02/2009). One might argue that he was being a 23-year-old with limited instincts of danger to his reputation and his fortune. He discounted the fact that somebody might take a photograph of him.

[8]Impulsivity is defined as (1) the inclination to choose small, immediately available rewards over larger, delayed rewards, and/or (2) the inclination to respond rapidly without forethought and/or attention to consequences.

[9]For example, a decision by a college student to buy an electronic item (iPod) impulsively, without thinking about the long-term consequences.

Addiction

Preference for short-term rather than longer-term rewards is a hallmark of substance abuse and other addictive behaviors. Research supports that delay discounting is a major factor contributing to the problem of drug abuse (Bickel et al., 2007). Addicts consistently show a greater preference for small, immediate rewards over larger, delayed rewards (e.g., money). This relationship is found in individuals who are nicotine-dependent, are opiate-dependent, or who use alcohol at high (problematic) levels (Bickel et al., 2007). For addicts, delayed outcomes appear to have little value. For example, smokers know that smoking may give lung cancer, and still smoke.

However, showed that ex-smokers of cigarettes discounted money no differently than nonsmokers. The finding suggests that either the degree of discounting decreases after abstinence is achieved or people who are more likely to achieve abstinence discount less steeply. Yoon et al. (2007) found that in women who had quit smoking during pregnancy, those with a higher degree of discounting were more likely to have relapsed to smoking by 6 months postpartum. Overall, these findings suggest that people who discount more sharply may be more likely to initiate smoking and subsequently unable to quit. Thus, steep discounting may provide a risk factor for drug use and addiction.

Cognitive Capacity

It is well established that cognitive[10] ability is a powerful predictor of success in life. Cognitive development is essential for information processing, learning, and decision making. Discounting represents a critical variable through which intelligence influences economic outcomes (Heckman, 2007). Discounting involves the "executive brain," which is linked to intelligence through the function of prefrontal cortex. Higher intelligence is associated with lower discounting. Children with higher intelligence tend to be better at shifting attention away from the affective properties of the rewards. They are also more adept at transforming reward representations to make them more abstract and, consequently, lower discounting.[11]

---

[10]According to the American Psychological Association Dictionary, cognition is defined as "all forms of knowing and awareness such as perceiving, conceiving, remembering, reasoning, judging, imagining, and problem solving".

[11]Professor Nisbett (2009) in is his book, "Intelligence and How to Get It," provides suggestions for improving I.Q. that include praising effort more than achievement and teaching youth delayed gratification.

This explains why individuals with lower intelligence may be more prone to financial hardships, and they tend to have lower levels of financial asset accumulation.

Time preferences are linked to the ability to imagine future states. Becker and Mulligan (1997) suggest that imagining the future more vividly can decrease our discount rate for that future. They argue that the discount rate is a function of the resources invested in imagining the future. They explain that decision makers maximize lifetime utility subject to difficulties in envisioning exactly how rewarding the future will be. Hence, people will expend resources to make their image of the future vivid and clear. For example, we might spend time with our parents to remind ourselves of what our needs will be when we are their age.

Moreover, the process of deciding whether to choose an immediate reward or a delayed but higher reward is strongly associated with success in life. Consider, for example, the classic research conducted by Walter Mischel and his colleagues at the Bing Nursery School at Stanford University. Preschoolers were given a choice between receiving a large reward (e.g., two marshmallows) on the return of the experimenter or, at any time during the delay, forgoing the larger reward by accepting a smaller but immediately available reward (e.g., one marshmallow). Their study demonstrates the children's ability to transform the "hot" thoughts associated with immediate gratification into "cool" ones. In a longitudinal follow-up, preschoolers' duration of waiting before selecting the smaller-sooner reward was predictive of academic and social competence in adolescence (Mischel, Shoda, & Peake, 1988). Preschoolers who waited longer were more likely than their more impulsive peers to become adolescents who more successfully coped with stress and frustration, demonstrated better abilities to concentrate and maintain attention, better responded to reason, and scored higher on the SAT. Thus, being smarter can also give us the ability to think more clearly about our goals, objectives, and values.

Cognitive Deficit[12]

Life is full of distractions. At a cognitive level, the ability to stay on a course depends on the functional integrity of the frontal lobes.[13] Being at the mercy of incidental distraction and displaying an inability to follow

---

[12]Scientists first began to gain an understanding of the role of the prefrontal cortex in 1848 with the case of Phineas Gage. Gage, a hardworking and conscientious railroad employee, was the victim of a freak accident in which an explosion drove a steel rod through his skull. Gage survived the accident but seemed to undergo an abrupt personality change.

plans are common features of frontal lobe disorders. When neurological illness affects the frontal lobes, the ability to stay on track becomes lost, and the patient is completely at the mercy of incidental distractions.[14] This syndrome is different than the proverbial "absent-minded professor," where cognitive overloading increases distractions in normal subjects.

Patients with orbitofrontal syndrome[15](due to head injury, brain disease, or dementia) are emotionally disinhibited. Their ability to inhibit the urge for instant gratification is severely impaired. They do what they feel like doing, without any concern for social taboos or legal prohibition (e.g., shoplifting, sexually aggressive behavior, or reckless driving). There is also disparity between knowledge and the ability to guide behavior with this knowledge. These patients will say the right things but make the wrong choices at the same time[16] (Goldberg, 2009).

Socioeconomic Characteristics

Wealthier individuals are more productive at producing future-oriented capital (education, saving, and health prevention). Poverty and the pressure of present needs blind a person to the needs of the future, thereby

---

(*cont.*) He retained his intelligence, but he was no longer sober and reliable. He could no longer conform his behavior to specific goals. Scientists now believe that the rod destroyed Gage's orbital prefrontal cortex, the part of the brain in charge of encoding goals and assigning relative value to them.

[13]In many cases the cognitive deficit takes very subtle forms, not apparent through simple observation. One test to detect this is known as the Stroop Test (**Blue Purple Red**), after the name of its inventor. It is one of the best-known tests of self-control. The subject is to look at a list of color names printed in discordant colors (e.g., word "blue" printed in red or the other way around) and to name the colors, instead of reading the words. The test requires that you resist your immediate impulse to read the word, which is the natural tendency of reading the printed material. It requires self-control to turn off our reading impulse and respond solely to the color of the actual letters.

[14]Attention deficit hyperactivity disorder (ADHD), with its extreme distractibility, is usually linked to frontal lobe dysfunction. His or her attention drifts on any task devoid of instant reward (a computer game or sporting event), such as listening to a lecture or reading a textbook.

[15]The syndrome is also known as ventromedial syndrome. Damasio (1994) demonstrates that patients with damage to the ventromedial prefrontal cortex (VMPF) lack social maturity for working within a social group. Within a social group, members have different goals and needs and are never in perfect agreement, and the capacity for compromise is a critical mechanism for social harmony. This capacity depends on our ability to control the negative emotions arising from an inability to find immediate gratification. Impulsive or opportunistic choices (e.g., taking advantage of one's friends) provide immediate positive outcome, whereas their negative consequences (e.g., jail, loss of friends) are discounted.

[16]Several years ago, an obstetrician carved his initial into a woman's belly after performing a C-section. Reportedly, the doctor said he felt that his surgery had been such a masterpiece that he had to sign it. As claimed by his lawyer, the doctor suffered from frontal lobe damage.

increasing time preference. For example, if your heat is about to shut off and there is no food in the house, you have more immediate concerns than the possible future poor health consequences of consuming French fries. In this case, poverty focuses individuals' attention on the present and decreases the value that they place on the future.

Delay discounting is also related to educational level. Better educated people will have lower discount rates. Education may enlighten people with regard to the value of deferred versus current consumption. People with more education tend to have a longer time horizon, and they are more likely to look at the long-term consequences of their health behavior. One possible explanation is that the affluent, well-educated population finds the future, especially the prospect of retirement, far more attractive than the lower-income population for whom the future means only continuing economic worries. Another explanation is that education raises cognition, which in turn improves behavior. Better educated people seem better at quitting bad habits or at controlling their consumption (Cutler et al., 2010). The better educated tend to be more successful in translating intentions into actions.[17] In short, education seems to influence cognitive ability, and cognitive ability in turn leads to healthier behaviors. The impact of cognitive ability is not so much about the level of information, but the way one processes information. People are generally informed about the negative consequences of poor nutrition and obesity, but the better educated may understand it better (Cutler, Lleras-Muney, & Vogl, 2010).

Anticipation (Pleasure of Expectation)

In contrast to the discounting model, the desire to reduce dread implies that people may prefer to endure a bad experience (like a trip to the dentist) earlier rather than later. The usual explanation for such behavior is that waiting for unpleasant outcomes induces anxiety that can be avoided by getting the outcomes over with quickly. Pleasant experiences, like vacations or dates, may be deliberately postponed or planned well ahead of time so they can be "savored." In general, people tend to derive pleasure from anticipating good things and discomfort from anticipating bad things.

---

[17]Alternatively, there may be some third factor that influences both education and health behaviors. Research suggests that education affects health because both are determined by individual differences in time preferences and the value people place on the future (Fuchs, 1986). Those who attach a low rate of time discounting tend to value education. It is also plausible that higher education may shape time preference in that direction.

Summary

People are not equally patient. They differ in their degree of discounting. For example, those who are younger, have low income, or are less intelligent may have higher discount rates. Discounting is a useful diagnostic tool and a key factor to design treatment strategies that will reduce addictions and manage impulsive behavior. Also, if people are taught to value delayed consequences in treatment, the learning could potentially generalize to other aspects of their lives.

Environments characterized by economic deterioration and destabilization, in which the future outcomes of one's behavior are typically characterized by risk and uncertainty, may encourage shortsighted behavior (Bickel & Johnson, 2003). The prevalence of substance abuse, overeating, criminal behavior, and many other types of risk behavior is higher in urban and low SES residential environments (Bickel et al., 2007). In many inner-city environments, where community instability and decay (e.g., poverty and violence) are endemic, considering one's future may seem a fruitless endeavor for individuals who may not expect to experience the future. In such a situation, the most adaptive strategy may be to consider exclusively the immediate consequences of a behavior.

HOW WE EVALUATE THE FUTURE

Individual differences in the way that people make trade-offs between present and future are captured by the notion of a discount rate, which is a function of when outcomes occur. In economics, a discount rate, or rate of return, captures one's preference for consuming earlier rather than later. This section briefly describes the standard approach for evaluating future rewards, followed by hyperbolic discounting to explain individual time-inconsistent behavior. Hyperbolic discounting shows that people devalue a given future event at different rates, depending on how far away it is.

The Discounted Utility (DU) Model

The discounted utility (DU) model[18] is standard in economics and business. The model multiplies an individual's utility or payoffs in each period

---

[18]The DU model was introduced by Paul Samuelson in 1937. The model's popularity is rooted in its simplicity and analytical usefulness. However, Paul Samuelson warned about its limited value in describing the way people discount the future.

by a weight that represents the individual's rate of time preference and aggregates the sum of the weighted utilities:

$$U(x) = \sum_{t=0}^{T} D(t)u(x_t),$$

where $U(x)$ is the discounted present value, $u(x_t)$ is the value or payoffs of some choice x at time t, and $D(t)$ is a discounting factor (not the same as discount rate). The discount factor is a weight that reflects the reduction in value of some commodity due to its delay. The higher the discount factor, the more the future is valued. The typical present value (PV) formulation uses two terms: the discount rate, r, and the discounting factor, $DF = (1/1 + r)^t$.

The following example illustrates the discounted value for three periods with various payoffs and discount rate of 8%. Normally, the project is acceptable if its PV exceeds the initial investment. The present value is often referred to as the indifferent point between accepting it now or waiting to receive it in the future.

t	DF	DF	Cash Flow	PV
0	1	1	150	150.00
1	1/1.08	0.93	100	93.00
2	1/(1.08)2	0.853	300	257.00
				PV = $500

Exponential Discount Function

In general, economists assume a discounting of future reward by a factor of $(1 + r)^{-t}$, where r is the constant discount rate per unit of time and t is the duration of delay. This is known as *exponential discounting*. The larger discount rate, the less the person cares about the future (a steeper function), and consequently the individual is acting in a more myopic manner.

For example, consider a benefit that will materialize in 20 years. If the value of that benefit is $20,000 (in dollars of constant purchasing power), at a discount rate of 5%, then its present value is $7,500 [(20,000 $\times$ 1/(1.05)^{20}]. At a discount rate of 15%, its present value is $1,200 [(20,000 $\times$ 1/(1.15)^{20}].

In the business world, savings banks offer compound interest. They calculate interest frequently, add it to the principal, and recalculate the next period's interest based on the total. For a given interest rate, as the frequency of compounding increases, actual interest approaches a maximum, expressed by the following (exponential) discount function: $V = Ae^{-rD}$ Where V = present value (now), A = delayed value (then), D = delay,

r = discount rate, e is the base of natural logarithms (about 2.72). For example, the discount rate (interest rate) is 5% per year and if the money were left in the bank for 20 years, rD would be equal 1.00. If A is $20,000, at a discount rate of 5% its present value, V, is $7,358 (20,000 $\times$ e$^{-1.00}$).

Consistent Behavior over Time

The exponential discounting model predicts consistency of preference over time. This is a standard assumption, used in economics, that a person's preferences does not change over time. If an individual prefers one apple today to two apples tomorrow, then he will prefer one apple in one year to two apples in a year and a day. In general, economically speaking a person's preference between two alternatives does not vary no matter when he evaluates them. Individuals who exhibit exponential discounting behavior when faced with a choice between a smaller/sooner (SS) reward or larger/later (LL) reward do not change their preference as the SS reward becomes present. Rather, such individuals continually choose options that maximize their total happiness with allowances for the reduced value of the delayed rewards. In the context of health behavior, exponential discounting implies a stability of preference over time; that is, resolutions once made are never broken (e.g., resolutions to quit smoking or stick to a diet are always carried out.)

This pattern is seen in Figure 6.1, the relative value of two future rewards remains the same as one moves closer toward them in time. The curves represent the present values of two rewards as evaluated at various earlier times.

Myopia and Rationality

Exponential discounting can be highly myopic without being inconsistent. It is important to note that for an economist, rationality resides in the form of the discount function and not in the interest rate itself. Rational

FIGURE 6.1 Exponential Discount Function

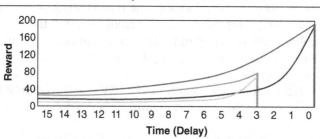

behavior means acting in a manner that is consistent with one's utility function. A person who discounts future rewards extremely, who prefers $10 today to $100 tomorrow, would be deemed myopic (shortsighted) by an economist. But if that person's preference were consistent (if the person preferred $10 tomorrow to $100 the day after tomorrow, $10 in 10 days to $100 in 11 days; in general, $10 in x days to $100 in $x + 1$ days), the economist would consider that person's preference to be perfectly rational. In other words, exponential discounting can be highly myopic without being inconsistent.

Economists argue that there are no such things as irrational preferences. In the same way that preferences for food items differ across people, so do preferences for time. Some people are much more focused on short-term gains than others: they base their decisions on a higher discount rate than other people. Thus, caring less about the future than the present can be rational. Some like apples, others like oranges; some like the present, others like the future. Thus, if a person discounts the future very heavily, consuming an addictive substance may, for him, be a form of rational behavior. Such a person with a consistently high discount rate does not experience internal conflict (self-control problem). So, a rational overeater or drug addict may have a problem, but it is not a self-control problem.[19]

Time Inconsistent Behavior (Hyperbolic Discounting)

Suppose you set your alarm clock at midnight to wake up at 6:00 A.M. the next day. At midnight it "seems sensible" to you to sleep 6 hours, get up at 6:00 A.M. and put in a full day of work. But when the alarm goes off the next morning, the choice that you made last night now seems absurd. This inconsistency rests on an illusion that we all experience. When we can hold all alternatives at a distance, our evaluation of them remain true to their values in our lives. But our subjective evaluation of a reward (our appetite for it) grows when we are closer to the reward than when we are far away, and unless we somehow commit ourselves to our previous preferences, we succumb. This tendency is often referred to as *hyperbolic discounting, present bias,* or time inconsistent behavior (Ainslie, 2001; Laibson, 1997). This change in preference is often the source of self-control problems. We often want instant gratification and want to be patient in the future, such as eating highly caloric foods while planning to diet starting tomorrow.

The hyperbolic formula is expressed as $PV = A/(1+rD)$, in which PV is the present value, A is the delayed reward, D is the delay, r is the discount

---

[19]As the saying goes, *everyone wants to go heaven, but nobody wants to die.*

rate, and higher r values are indicative of higher impulsivity. The addition of 1 prevents PV from becoming infinity at $t = 0$, when there is no delay. This formula says that the discounted present value of 1 unit of benefit (utility) t periods into the future equals $1/(1 + rt)$.

For example, assume $r = 1$, and the person at $t = 0$ faces the choice between a reward of $10 at $t = 5$ and a reward of $30 at $t = 10$. At $t = 0$, the present value of the former is $1.67 and that of the latter is $2.73. A person who maximizes present value will choose the delayed reward. At $t = 1$, the present value of the earlier reward is 2 and that of the latter is 3. At $t = 2$, the values are 2.5 and 3.3; at $t = 3$, they are 3.3 and 3.75; and at $t = 4$, they are 5 and 4.29. At some time between $t = 3$ and $t = 4$, that is, the earlier reward becomes the most preferred option as we get closer to the reward.

$V[(1/(1 + r_i)]$	$PV(10), t = 5$	$PV(30), t = 10$
$T = 0$	10(1/6) = 1.667	30(1/11) = 2.73
$T = 1$	10(1/5) = 2	30(1/10) = 3
$T = 2$	2.5	3.3
$T = 3$	3.3	3.75
$T = 4$	5	4.29

Suppose the individual lowers the value of discount rate from 1 to 0.3 (by improving self-control). Now, at the time the smaller reward becomes available, its present value is simply 10 (no discounting), but the present value of the larger reward is 12 [$30/(1 + 0.3\times5)$, or $30/2.50$]. Thus, improving self-control enables this person to act in accordance with his calm and reflective judgment.

As Figure 6.2 demonstrates, hyperbolic discount functions decay at a more rapid rate in the short run than in the long run. So, a hyperbolic discounter is more impatient when making short-run trade-offs than when making long-run trade-offs.

The objective values of A and B are indicated by the height of the reward curve at point t_A and t_B that will be received in the future; their present values are decreased as the current time is approached. At time t_1, the larger reward (B) is preferred. However, at time t_2, the smaller reward (A) is preferred.

Summary

Standard economic theory suggests that each individual has a constant rate of time preference, and the rate is not context dependent. Alternatively, time preference is characterized by a hyperbolic functional

FIGURE 6.2   Preference Reversal

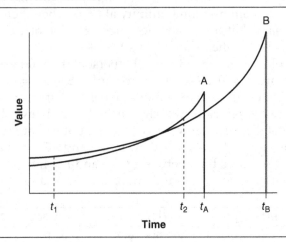

form, rendering short-term impulses supreme over long-term goals (Laibson, 1997). In contrast, behavioral economics research has shown that rates of time preference are not constant rates that result in exponential discounting, but, instead, vary by the time horizon faced. According to the model, individuals underestimate their future impulsivity, resulting in preference reversal as time passes.

The hyperbolic discounting model, or present-biased preference, predicts that individuals act irrationally in that they excessively discount the future. They favor long-run maximization at all times except as smaller rewards becomes more immediately available. Consequently, they often end up acting against their own best interest. They do worse in life because they spend too much for what they want now at the expense of goodies they want in the future. People buy things they cannot afford with credit cards, and as a result they get to buy less over the course of their lifetimes. The model underlies several socially important human behaviors, such as drug addiction, obesity, and unsafe sex. As discussed in Chapter 11, to counter these self-control problems, sophisticated agents employ commitment devices to attempt to protect long-term goals from short-term consumption decisions.

EXPLAINING EXCESSIVE CONSUMPTION

Heyman (2009) describes two frames of mind (local and global) in making decision. A *local choice perspective* refers to choosing between the available items one at a time. In a *global choice perspective*, we organize the items into sequences and then choose between different sequences. For example, deciding on what to eat at your nightly meal is the local approach. However, deciding between sequences of meals for a week is the global approach. With a local choice perspective, choosing the better option means choosing the item that currently has the highest value. With a global perspective, the best choice is the collection or sequence of items that has higher value.

The hyperbolic model is consistent with a local approach to decision making that leads to excessive consumption. The global choice is consistent with the rational economic model. For instance, when planning for the long term, most people intend to eat healthy foods, exercise regularly, watch less television, and quit smoking. They take a global perspective. But such plans require gratification to be delayed. Since on any given day the value of the current indulgence is always higher than the value of any distant health benefit, people tend to put off doing anything about their long-terms goals. However, when they regret their past behavior, they are taking a global perspective.

For a more practical example of how the model operates, consider someone who wants to start an exercise program but does not like to exercise. The exercise program entails, say, an immediate cost of eight units of value, but will produce a delayed benefit of 10 units. That is a net gain of two units, but it ignores the adjustment for the future value. If future events have perhaps half the value of present ones, then the 10 units become only five, and starting an exercise program today means a net *loss* of three units (8 − 5). So we are reluctant to start exercising *today*. On the other hand, starting *tomorrow* devalues both the cost *and* the benefit by half (to four and five units, respectively), resulting in a net *gain* of one unit from exercising. Hence, everyone is enthusiastic about going to the gym *tomorrow*. By the logic of hyperbolic discounting, this example illustrates that if the decision (local perspective) to go to the gym is made each morning at 6 A.M., and this person prefers an extra hour of sleep. He will plan to sleep just one more time and then start going to gym. Tomorrow, the same reasoning will apply. However, the global perspective will motivate one to focus on a pattern of lifestyle choice. Similarly, someone who has a second helping of dessert every night ends up 20 pounds heavier than he or she had planned. Thus, health behavior choices that create an undesirable way of life are made one day at a time. They are not made at the level of a lifestyle.

This is because the rewards associated with the global perspective accrue rather slowly. At the beginning of a period of abstinence from drugs, for example, the pleasure of a day of sobriety is less than the value of the most recent drug day. On a daily basis, the cost (pain) of abstinence exceeds its benefits. From a local choice, quitting can only occur if there is a change in conditions that markedly reduces the value (pleasure) of the drug relative to the nondrug alternative. This means that quitting requires a steadfast commitment to the global approach to choice and a plan of action that erases reminders of the day-to-day pleasures of drug use.

Relapse

Why is relapse so often preceded by the statement that this is a "special occasion?" And why is a "special occasion" a good excuse to have another drink? The excuse reflects an underlying dilemma. From a local perspective, the drug is the best choice; but from a global perspective, abstinence is the best choice. The ideal solution is to somehow do both. This is impossible, except in one situation. If the situation can be framed as the "last time," then the dilemma dissolves, since the person can say to himself or herself that a new and better life will begin tomorrow.

On any occasion, overeating produces limited harm. The damage occurs after repeated indulgences. Thus, the focus of treatment should be less on the individual occasion of impulse control. The better solution arises from reframing the problem such that failure in any occasion is a predictor of failure in all occasions. If I give in today, I shall fail tomorrow as well. By connecting these single occasions into a sequence and thus raising the stakes, the individual can gain a motivation to control his or her impulses that would be lacking if he or she just considers one day at the time.

THE ROLE OF TIME PREFERENCE IN OBESITY

A body of research shows that obese individuals (especially women) have higher rates of discounting (i.e., are more impulsive) (Davis et al., 2007). This suggests that obese individuals make more impulsive food-related decisions compared with individuals of normal weight (Weller, Cook, Avsar, & Cox, 2008). Factors that influence impulsive decision making are fundamental to obesity treatment and prevention efforts. For example, the increased prevalence of obesity is linked to ready access to inexpensive, high-calorie foods. These food alternatives may compete with delayed, possibly healthier meals made at home. Thus, in advanced countries, where the costs of caloric intake in terms of both money and time are so low, those with less patience would tend to have higher BMI values and a higher probability of being obese (Scharff, 2009; Smith, Bogin, & Bishai, 2005). For example, Cutler, Glaeser, and Shapiro (2003) suggest that those with self-control problems are more likely to have high initial weight levels and are more likely to gain more weight with improvements in food technology.

Hyperbolic discounting leads people to please their immediate appetite and eat excessively cheap, fatty foods. Consider, for example, the role of food assistance programs on nutrient intake and body weight. Shapiro (2005) shows that participants in low-income families who were provided food stamps by the U.S. government displayed eating behaviors that are consistent with hyperbolic discounting. Because food stamp benefits are paid once a month, recipients may find themselves in a cycle of food deprivation at the end of the month followed by increased intake of comforting, high-calorie food, and binge eating when their benefits arrive. The study showed that participants tend to shift expenditures to cheaper foods as the month progresses. In particular, Shapiro revealed that food stamp recipients exhibit impatience by consuming more calories at the beginning of the food stamp cycle than at the end of the cycle.

The presence of hyperbolic discounting in food consumption decisions suggests that providing nutrition information (through labeling and targeted educational programs) is a necessary, but not sufficient, condition for optimal consumer decision making. Policymakers must find ways to help consumers deal with the self-control problems associated with hyperbolic discounting. For example, the presence of hyperbolic discounting suggests that the most effective commitment mechanisms will transfer the present value of the long-term costs of obesity closer to the point of consumption.[20] Policies that raise the immediate costs of choices that lead to obesity are likely to be effective at reducing the prevalence of obesity. For example, a sin tax on unhealthy foods would directly raise the present costs of being obese in the future, and thereby suppress the obesity rate. Similarly, policies that aim at educating people to be more future-oriented, or providing incentives for them to use precommitment devices, might yield higher returns to current investment. Policies that ease self-control problems are also likely to be effective. For example, by conducting field experiments in fast food restaurants, Downs, Loewenstein, and Wisdom (2009) report that consumers' calorie intake is reduced by arranging the menu so that the front page contains only low-calorie food. In sum, consumers operating with hyperbolic preferences must not only be educated about the risks they face and how to eat more healthfully but also be taught to overcome their temporally inconsistent preferences through the use of commitment mechanisms.

The relationship between time preference and obesity is potentially important because an individual's intertemporal choice could be the ultimate culprit of most behaviors that lead to obesity (e.g., adopting

---

[20]For example, while a small weight gain may not be visually noticeable, the weekly Weight Watchers weigh-in forces an individual to confront the implications of his or her consumption on a weekly basis.

a sedative lifestyle or eating compulsively). For instance, most weight control methods require one to forgo current consumption of unhealthy foods in order to reap future health gains. Hence, individuals who want to lose weight but lack the willpower will find it more difficult to stick to their diet and exercise plans, leaving them at a higher risk for obesity.

CONCLUSION

Health behavior choices, such as overeating and substance use, involve a tension between a desire for immediate gratification and delayed gratification. This chapter showed that the combination of individual and environmental forces influence the host of vulnerability for temporal discounting. In the language of public health, a genetic predisposition for extreme temporal discounting could be considered as a risk factor. Thus, promoting consideration of the future consequences of behavior may be an important policy tool to improve human well-being.

7

How We Make Decisions: The Role of Emotion

INTRODUCTION

How do we make decisions? And how can we improve our decision making? Understanding the way people make decisions dramatically increases our capacities for practical self-control and helps to design strategies to promote healthy behavior.

The standard approach to decision making is the concept of rational choice as discussed in any typical microeconomics textbooks. Decision makers are assumed to consciously weigh the potential consequences of their decisions dispassionately and to choose options that maximize total happiness. According to the rational model, when we are deciding what to do, we are able to ignore our feelings and carefully think through the options. In fact, emotion is viewed as a negative influence and obstacle to the rational decision-making process. However, evidence is accumulating in psychology and neuroscience that emotions and rational thinking are closely intertwined. The findings point out that emotions interfere with rational decision making by affecting both the cognitive and the motivational forces that shape decisions.

This chapter describes the relevance of emotion to understanding individual decision making. It will show that individual behavior is the outcome of an interaction between a deliberative system and an emotion system that operate according to different principles and often clash with one another. The final decision is determined by the relative strength of emotional and reflective forces. The relative contribution of emotion and reflective processes depends on a number of circumstances. More specifically, this chapter will address (1) the interplay of emotions and cognition concerning the nature of decision making, (2) various factors that influence affective and reflective systems, (3) how these systems may transform into behavior, (4) what happens when they conflict with each other, and (5) how such conflicts among affective and cognitive determinants of action are resolved.

This chapter demonstrates the importance of integrating the role of emotion in individual decision making in light of current scientific understanding of the brain and its processes. Explaining the role of emotions in decision making contributes to more accurate view of individual behavior than the traditional model of rational choice. Advances in the neurobiological study of emotions suggest that thoughts and emotions are equally important to our behavior and the study of either one alone will be incomplete. The insight may account for seemingly inconsistent or irrational behaviors, such as impulsivity, overeating, and drug addiction. Finally, the chapter presents a framework that is also valuable for understanding decisions for our professional life, business life, and the way we look at the world.

THE DUAL MIND

At the basic level, the brain can be divided into the *neocortex*, the outer surface of the brain, and the deeper, evolutionarily older subcortical structures (below the cortex) that include the striatum (near the brain's core) and the brain stem (at its base). The "old brain"[1] was built on simple stimulus-response principles: if an apple smelled good and you were hungry, you ate it. The primitive, emotional parts of our brains interact with our modern cortexes to influence the choices we make.

Dual-process routes to behavior (e.g., cognition and emotion, reason and intuition, or consciousness and unconsciousness) are pervasive in contemporary psychology and neuroscience (Evans, 2008). In the economics and decision-making literatures, a distinction has been made between System 1 and System 2 mechanisms (Kahneman, 2003). System 1 corresponds closely to automatic processing, and System 2 corresponds closely to controlled processing. System 1 quickly proposes answers to problems as they arise, and System 2 monitors the quality of answers provided by System 1 and, in some situations, corrects or overrides these judgments.

For example, most Americans have an automatic response to a distance given in miles but have to use their cognitive system to process a distance in kilometers. But, for Europeans, the opposite is true. Emotion is explicitly linked to the System 1, whereas reflective decision making seems much more like a System 2 process. These dual-system models show that in making decisions, we seem to have two minds in one brain or a brain at war with itself (Stanovich, 2004). Examples include compulsive behaviors such as overeating, gambling, or smoking, where we may

---

[1] Many of our sufferings have to do with the mismatch between our old brain and the modern world in which we live. Obesity is a simple example. For most of human history, food was hard to get. In a world in which food is scarce, it is smart to eat whenever possible and store up the fat. But many humans now live in environments in which food is cheap, plentiful, and tasteful.

become aware of a System 1 and 2 conflict. We may judge these behaviors to be irrational because we compulsively behave in ways that are at odds with our explicitly stated (System 2) goals.

Neuroscientists also have proposed a similar distinction. For example, Bernheim and Rangel (2003) have hypothesized that the brain can operate in one of two modes, a "cold mode" or a "hot mode." In the cold mode, the person makes deliberative decisions with a broad, long-term perspective. In the hot mode, a person's decision making is influenced by emotions and motivational drives. Which mode is triggered depends on environmental cues, which in turn might depend on past behavior (e.g., the experience of craving for chocolate cake at a birthday party).

The neocortex (the CEO of the brain) plays the leading role in characterizing the options available and their consequences, whereas the emotional brain evaluates these options. The emotional brain is the home of preferences, whereas the neocortex improves the quality of decision making. With its help, we can make plans, we can postpone action, we can regulate our emotions, and we can imagine things that do not exist. Science, literature, philosophy, and religion could not have taken shape without it.

Therefore, individual decisions are best understood as the interactions between cognition and emotion, and these two systems coexist as independent entities (Loewenstein & O'Donoghue, 2004).[2] The deliberative system allows people to think about long-term goals and thereby escape temptation. The deliberative system can weigh long-term health risks against present pleasures, even though the emotion system has a hard time imagining the future. For example, our emotion system wants to order dessert and smoke a cigarette, and our deliberative brain knows we should resist the temptation and quit smoking. The final decision is determined by the relative strengths of these two systems. The final decision also depends on the compatibility of the two systems. If the two systems cooperate, the behavior is facilitated. However, the two systems may also compete, which is accompanied by a feeling of conflict and temptation. For example, a person who is on a diet may be tempted to eat a second desert, while, at the same time, the cognitive system generates a behavioral decision to refrain from eating. Table 7.1, adapted from Epstein, compares these modes of thought. In general, the *intuitive system* involves unconscious desires, relies on past experiences, is emotional, and relies on intuitions in making decisions. In contrast, the

---

[2]Psychologist John Haidt describes the dual model by the metaphor of the elephant and the rider. The affective system is like a great big and determined elephant. The reflective system is the rider sitting on the top with rather limited control. The elephant (affective system) is not easy to control, as we may want to.

TABLE 7.1   Two Ways of Thinking

Intuitive System (S1)	Analytic System (S2)
Uncontrolled	Controlled
Generalized: conducive to stereotypes	Analytic: discourages overgeneralization
Emotional: attuned to what feels good	Logical: based on what is sensible
Intuitive	Explicit
Impulsive	Reflective
Low effort	High effort
Associative—mediated by vibes from past experience	Deductive—mediated by conscious appraisal of events
Rapid	Slow
Holistic	Analytic
High capacity	Low capacity
Skilled	Rule-following
Self-evident: "seeing is believing"	Requires justification via logic and evidence
Default process	Inhibitory
Unconscious	Conscious

Source: Adapted from Epstein (1994).

analytic system uses conscious and deliberate cognitive processes to make decisions. The intuitive system processes many things simultaneously and often unconsciously (e.g., speaking in your native language and craving chocolate). The reflective system has limited capacity, but offers more systematic analysis (e.g., learning a new language and counting calories).

THE DELIBERATIVE–AFFECTIVE MODEL

This section describes a framework in which a person's decision is the outcome of an interaction between deliberative and affective systems.[3] The discussion illustrates the mechanisms through which these systems exert their joint influence on the individual decisions. The two systems use different operations. The affective system is primarily driven by motivational mechanisms and the deliberative system takes into account broader goals (Loewenstein & O'Donoghue, 2004).

---

[3]The idea of a division between affective and deliberative systems appears as early as in the discussions of Greek philosophers under the labels of passion and reason. They argued that people act against their better judgment when they are overpowered by their passions. The idea of reason is generally connected to impartiality, such as the desire to promote the public good rather than private ends, or concern with long-term interest rather than short-term concern.

The term *affect* is an umbrella term that encompasses emotions,[4] mood, and drive states (e.g., hunger, thirst, sex, and pain). All affects carry "action tendencies," such as anger motivates us to take action, pain to take steps to ease the pain, and fear to escape or freeze. The affective processes are those that address "go/no-go" questions and motivate approach or avoidance behavior.

The deliberative system tends to be invoked deliberately and is often associated with a subjective feeling of effort. Because deliberate processing is conscious, people often have reasonably good introspective access to it. If students are asked how they solved a math problem or chose a new car, they can often provide a fairly accurate account of their choice process.[5] By contrast, when it comes to emotional reactions, a person may not be able to give a more satisfying explanation of an action except that "he felt like it."

Many decision-making disorders may originate in an improper division of labor between the systems. The decisions of an impulsive individual are excessively influenced by external stimuli, pressures, and demands. By contrast, an obsessive-compulsive person will subject even the most trivial decisions to extensive deliberation and cost-benefit calculation. In situations in which it is entirely appropriate to make a quick decision (e.g., a video rental), the obsessive-compulsive will get stuck. Under certain circumstances, the affective system prevails, and people succumb to things such as drug addiction and overeating. When the deliberative system is damaged, then the affective system loses its restraint (Bechara & Damasio, 2005). Thus, our desire and emotions are immune to the power of reason.

Figure 7.1 graphically represents the dual model that integrates the role of both emotion and cognition in determining behavior. There is a bidirectional link between these two processes to indicate the mutual influence that they have on each other. The model is a simplistic but heuristically powerful way to explain the organization of the brain. The intention is to convey the idea that behavior is the outcome of an interaction between distinct affective and deliberative systems.[6] The brain

---

[4]Emotion is movement. The word *emotion* comes from a Latin word that means "to move" or "to stir up." Emotion is also described as "a physiological" departure from homeostasis that it is subjectively experienced as a strong feeling (as of love, hate, or fear) and manifests itself in bodily changes. Emotional behavior strongly suggests a certain prominence of urges to act. For example, one in love or addiction tends to do certain things knowing the negative consequences.

[5]Standard tools of economics, such as a decision when you deliberate whether to buy a new car, represent deliberate processes. Thus, economics captures the parts of this process.

[6]Neurobiologists argue that the two-system model is inadequate, and they note that decisions are determined by the interactions of various brain systems.

FIGURE 7.1   The Two-System Model of Making Decisions

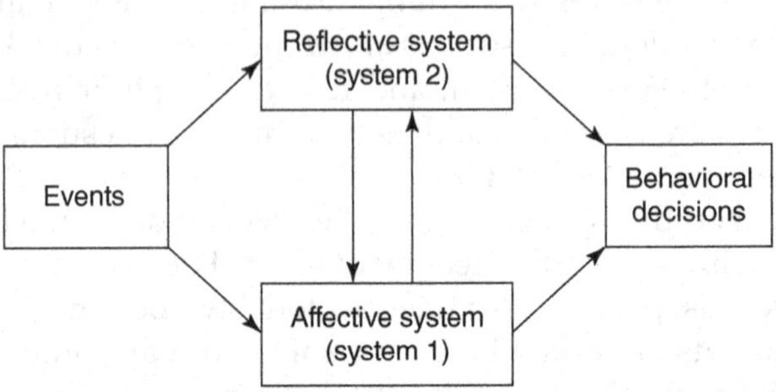

region that supports emotion and the brain region that supports cognition are completely intertwined. Every region in the brain that has been identified with some aspect of emotion has also been identified with aspects of cognition processes (Davidson & Irwin, 1999).

INFLUENCING FACTORS

What will eventually control a behavior depends on both situational and personal factors that moderate the relative strength of emotion and reflective forces. The following sections describe the factors that enhance the activation of the emotion and deliberative systems.

Stimuli

An environmental stimulus might activate the affective system, as when the sight of a delicious food motivates you to eat, or it might activate the deliberative system to remind you that you are on a diet. In fact, many stimuli activate both systems. For example, the sight of food activates the affective state of hunger and the cognitive state of "it's time to have lunch."

Stimuli are assumed to trigger the affective system through conditioning. For example, chronic exposure to highly palatable foods or drug use changes our brains, conditioning us to seek continued stimulation. Environmental cues are paired in time with an individual's consumption and, through classical conditioning, take on conditioned stimulus properties. When those cues are present at a later time, they elicit anticipation of a reward and thus generate craving. The learned cues capture our attention and motivate us to act. Cues can gain power even if we are not consciously aware of them. Over time, repeated responses to a salient cue followed by immediate reward strengthens the association between the cue and its reward. Most importantly, affective processes of behavior determination operate in an effortless manner.

The Role of Proximity

The proximity of a stimulus exerts a powerful influence on the affective system. Proximity can be defined on many dimensions, such as geographic, temporal, visual, social, and so forth. For example, a tasty food is more likely to evoke hunger to the extent that it is nearby, easily available, visible, or being consumed by someone else (in close proximity). Likewise, we are less influenced by celebrities' body types in the media than the appearance of the very real people to whom we are actually connected.

Perhaps the best evidence on the role of proximity comes from a series of classic studies conducted by Walter Mischel and Ayduk (2004). Young subjects (ages 4–13) were instructed by an experimenter that they could have a snack immediately or they could have a larger snack if they waited for the experimenter to return. The experimenter then measured how long the subjects were willing and able to wait for the larger snack (with a cap of 15 minutes). The experiment demonstrated that the child's ability to wait depended crucially on whether the inferior prize (the smaller snack) was visible. Merely covering the snack significantly enhanced the child's ability to wait. This behavior is consistent with the hypothesis that seeing the candy triggers strong visceral states (cravings), during which the child's thoughts are restricted to a limited range of activities and outcomes.

In short, emotions are highly tuned to temporal proximity. The affective systems kick in when rewards and punishments are immediate but not when they are remote. Deliberation is, in contrast, much less sensitive to immediacy.

The Vividness Effect

The affective system is highly attuned to visual imagery, whereas the deliberative system is much more keyed into the logic of costs and benefits. Abstract information generally has weak impact, compared with the impact of pictures and of events actually seen.[7]

Research shows that imagining our emotional reactions, or our anticipated emotions, increases the urge to act (McGaugh, 2003). For example, imagining one's satisfaction from eating chocolate cake may undermine the deliberative system by making the taste and smell of the cake more

---

[7]For example, teaching the hardship of parenting, a school program provides teenagers with dolls that require constant attention. The rationale is that, absent such a vivid experience, teenagers may have an overly romantic view of parenting, even if they are provided with more detailed information about the demands of parenting.

vivid in one's imagination. Activation of these vivid attributes may become so salient that they outweigh other factors (e.g., weight gain, calories, or fat content). Thus, individuals faced with a desirable stimulus may overweigh the impact of joy from satisfying the impulse compared with the guilt associated with failure to control the impulse.

The effect can be used to reverse behavior. Consider the use of vividness effect in the case of an antiobesity ad, which ran in New York. The ad shows a soda bottle which pours out thick, yellow human fat, mixed with blood vessels. It is accompanied by the words "Are you pouring on the pounds?" The image is designed to give people a shock and to raise the awareness about the billions of hidden calories, which Americans consume each year in sodas and other sugary drinks. However, the critics argue that shock advertising can backfire. They note that these images look so disgusting that some people might look away without paying attention to the message.

Time Pressure

Because deliberation is slow, deliberative processing takes time. Hence, any factor that imposes time pressure on a judgment or decision will tend to undermine deliberative processing. Under time pressure, people fall back on old habits (e.g., snacking on chips) even when they are not the desired response. With sufficient time to think, people are able to correct their gut-level response.[8]

THE INTERPLAY OF AFFECT AND COGNITION

Cognitive processes influence affect. Emotional reaction to a stimulus is not necessarily, or even usually, a reflex action, but often involves an appraisal of surrounding conditions. According to *appraisal theory*, emotional reaction is a function of private interpretation of an event. For example, consider a case of an employee suffering from depression. When asked what is going on in her life, she responds that her supervisor had recently given her an impossible task to complete and had berated her

---

[8]Psychologist Alison Lenton and economist Marco Francesconi illustrated the role of time pressure in speed dating (Lenton & Francesconi, 2010). They analyzed records from 84 different speed dating events held in bars and clubs across the United Kingdom. Speed dating involves lots of choices within limited time (3–5 minutes). The result showed that when people have too many romantic choices, they tend to choose partners based on superficial physical characteristics and ignore attributes such as education, smoking status, and occupation.

when the results were not to his liking. Appraisal theory suggests that her depression is partly triggered by the fact that she blamed herself for her supervisor's poor communication and managerial skills. The feelings that result from this assessment direct action. Appraisals can be either conscious or unconscious. The concept of appraisal provides insights into the individual differences in emotion reactions.

The affective system can influence the deliberative system and often distort our thinking about the consequences of the behavior. Emotions change how we see the world and how we interpret the actions of others. Such input from the affective system may be required for sound deliberative thinking. The input from the affective system may help focus the deliberative system on relevant bodily needs. For example, when the affective system transmits hunger up to the deliberative system, it helps focus the deliberative system on the decision whether to eat. Affect can also distort and disrupt deliberative processing in various ways. Under the influence of powerful emotions, people are ready to believe almost anything. For example, people who are desperately ill, or whose children are ill, are often ready to embrace quack remedies, contrary to all scientific evidence.

Why are placebos are so effective? Medical studies have shown that placebos (which have no actual medical value) can be fairly effective against a wide variety of diseases, such as heart problems, depression, and ulcers. In short, they are effective because people believe in them. It is estimated that between 35% and 75% of people get better after receiving sugar pills (Waber et al., 2008). For example, in a study to test the efficacy of new painkiller, almost all the participants experienced pain relief from the pill when they were told it cost $2.50. But when the price was dropped to 10 cents, only half of them did (Ariely, 2008).

Two mechanisms are at work here. One is the belief and confidence or faith in the drug. The placebo effect depends on the prefrontal cortex. When people are told that they just received pain reliever medicine, their reflective brain responds by inhibiting the activity of their emotional brain that normally responds to pain. People *expect* to experience less pain, so they indeed do end up experiencing less pain. Their expectation becomes a self-fulfilling prophesy. Sometimes the fact that a doctor or nurse is paying attention to us and reassuring us not only makes us feel better but also triggers our internal healing processes.

The second mechanism is conditioning. The prefrontal cortex impacts brain stem regions linked to the opiate release, which in turn reduces the pain. Thus, in the case of pain, expectation can unleash hormones and neurotransmitters, such as endorphins and opiates, that not only block agony but produce exuberant highs. So, beware of the perception of value that can become of real value.

Collaboration and Competition

In the case of *collaboration between cognition and emotion,* negative emotions breed negative thoughts, which in turn trigger negative feelings. For example, when a person is hungry, he or she has a greater appetite for food. The "thought" of food exacerbates the state of hunger. Therefore, the final decision of how much food to buy is altered by the hunger state itself and the cognition, so that the person is likely to over estimate the amount of food needed.

Under many circumstances, the behavioral choice activated by the affective and the reflective systems, respectively, may conflict with each other. Which process wins out over the other in these cases will depend on the relative strength of affect and cognition. For instance, when a person is standing in the supermarket checkout line, the sight of a chocolate bar may activate the affective system to purchase it. Meanwhile, the reflective system may generate a behavioral decision to stop the purchase due to weight concerns. Such a struggle between incompatible behaviors by the affective and the reflective system is often accompanied by a feeling of internal conflict or temptation that characterizes many impulsive decisions.

The extent of collaboration and competition between cognitive and affective systems, and the outcome of conflict when it occurs, depends critically on the intensity of affect. At low levels of intensity, affect appears to play a largely "information" role (e.g., affect-as-information theory[9]). At intermediate levels of intensity, people begin to become conscious of conflicts between cognitive and affective inputs. Finally, at even greater levels of intensity, people often report themselves as being "out of control" or "acting against their own self-interest." This is a moment that we are least motivated to use the reflective system (Kirby & Guastello, 2001). Extreme fear produces panic and immobilization rather than effective escape. Uncontrolled anger toward another person can lead to behaviors, such as crimes of passion, that often end up doing the most damage to one's self. Thus, hyperactivity of the affective system can overwhelm or "hijack" the influence of the reflective system.

The Primacy of Affect

Although interactions run in both directions, affect seems to hold a kind of primacy over deliberation; it is "first on the scene" and plays a dominant role in behavior. Anyone who has ever been put in front

---

[9]Central to the affect-as-information logic is the assumption that people draw on their affective experiences as a source of information. To make decisions, people may consciously inspect their feelings to see "how they feel" about the options. For example, when selecting a video, one considers various choices until one of them feels right (e.g., "would I have fun watching this movie?").

of a table of snacks and who has found himself eating without having made any deliberation can appreciate this notion.

There are many more neural connections going from the emotional systems to the deliberative systems than the other way. According to LeDoux (1996), while conscious control over emotions is weak, emotions can flood consciousness. This is so because the connections from the emotional systems to the cognitive systems are stronger than connections from the cognitive systems to the emotional systems. Evidence suggests that some people (e.g., aggressive people) tend to have a less active prefrontal lobe in general (Goldberg, 2009).

Automatic priming is a good example of the primacy of affect. Priming exerts an automatic effect on individuals' behavior. Exposure to hot affective cues triggers automatic action initiation. For example, in a study exposed customers in a supermarket drinks section to either French music or German music. The results showed that French wine outsold German wine when French music was played, whereas German wine outsold French wine when German music was played. However, the majority of customers denied that type of music playing influenced their choice of wine. Similarly, large portion sizes can prime food consumption, presumably because larger amounts highlight the tempting features of food and reduce people's capacity to consciously monitor the amount they have eaten.

THE ROLE OF WILLPOWER

An important aspect of being human is the ability to engage in reflective, controlled behavior (Higgins, 1996). Although the emotion system seems to hold primacy, the deliberative system can often override affective responses (at least partially). The existence of neural connections from the prefrontal cortex to the affective system suggests that the deliberative system can influence the affective system. The reflective system allows the individuals to make flexible decisions, proving a fairly large degree of control over choices and action. Rollo May (1981) defines freedom as the pause between stimulus and response. When we pause, we become free; we are no longer a part of the automatic reaction.

The efforts by the deliberative system to override affective motivations require an inner exertion of effort, often referred to as *willpower* (Baumeister, 2002). In general, willpower refers to effortful control that is exerted with the purpose of controlling our behavior. Willpower operates within the broader domain of *self-regulation*, defined as the process of controlling thoughts, behavior, attention, and emotions to achieve a personally desirable goal. When people exercise willpower or self-regulation, they inhibit their normal, typical, or automatic behavior. For example, if someone typically drinks sodas with meals, then it requires the exertion of willpower to alter this habit.

Willpower strength (or self-regulatory resources) fuels the reflective system. Low self-regulatory resource levels disable reflective activation, and hence the impulsive system will have a greater influence on behavior. However, willpower strength is a limited resource. Like any other limited resource, it is subject to the law of diminishing returns. Once the strength is used up, the reflective system becomes vulnerable. For instance, after resisting the temptation to eat freshly baked cookies, participants in one study quit sooner on a subsequent task requiring effortful persistence, compared with participants who did not have to resist eating the cookies. Resisting the temptation to eat the cookies presumably depleted an energy resource that could otherwise have been used to persist on the subsequent task (Baumeister, 2002).

Similarly, making many decisions leaves a person in a depleted state and less likely to exert willpower. When resources are depleted, people tend to make poor choices and are more likely to be swayed by desires, urges, and cravings, although they may regret them in the long run. Depleted persons succumb to various flawed decision strategies, by taking short cuts instead of reasoning out the problem. The following describes several factors that deplete willpower.

Cognitive Load

An important function served by the prefrontal cortex is what is called "working memory." It enables us to hold small amounts of information, such as a phone number, in mind for short periods of time. *Cognitive overload* can occur when there are too many tasks competing for finite cognitive resources. Research has shown that cognitive overload undermines efforts at self-control. For example, Shiv and Fedorikhin (1999) asked respondents to memorize either a two-digit number (low cognitive demand) or a seven-digit number (high cognitive demand). They were then asked to walk to another room to report this number. On the way, they were offered a choice between two snacks, chocolate cake (more favorable affect, less favorable cognitions) or fruit salad (less favorable affect, more favorable cognitions). The researchers predicted that the condition with high-memory load (seven digits) would reduce the capacity for deliberation, thus increasing the likelihood that the more emotionally favorable option (cake) would be selected. The prediction was confirmed. Chocolate cake was selected 63% of the time when the cognitive/memory load was high and only 41% of the time when memory load was low. Why did the two groups behave so differently? The effort to memorize seven digits drew cognitive resources away from the part of the brain that normally controls emotional urges.[10]

Ego Depletion

Because all acts of volition and self-control are effortful, making choices results in a state of *ego depletion*. Ego depletion is a temporary reduction in the self's capacity. The proliferation of choice is associated with distress, resulting in what Schwartz (2004) refers to as "the tyranny of freedom" and shows how too many choices can be draining and confusing.[11] Making many choices (e.g., making a bridal registry, choosing college courses) impairs subsequent self-control (i.e., less physical stamina, reduced persistence in the face of failure, more procrastination). In short, ego depletion makes people think less intelligently. There is a personal price to choosing. Ego depletion also may explain why successful attempts to control one's bad habits often lead to substitution toward other unrelated bad habits.

Loneliness and Social Exclusion

Feeling socially excluded can get in the way of our ability to think clearly and exercise self-control. In one study, participants who were made to feel socially disconnected consumed, on average, more cookies (roughly twice as many) than those who were primed to feel socially accepted (DeWall, 2009). Is there any wonder that we turn to ice cream or other fatty foods when we are sitting at home feeling all alone in the world? We want to sooth the pain we feel by injecting sugar and fat content to the brain's pleasure center. Cacioppo and Partick (2008) note that impaired self-regulation stems from a fear rooted in each of us being helplessly and dangerously alone. This loss of willpower also helps explain the often observed tendency of rejected lovers to do things they later regret (Baumeister, DeWall, Ciarocco, & Twenge, 2005). In short, individuals

---

[10]Scientists are discovering that multitasking (keeping brains busy with digital inputs) does not condition people to learn better and remember information, or generate new ideas. For example, people experience better mood and learn better after a walk in nature than after a walk in a dense urban environment. Because processing a vast amount of information can make them mentally fatigued. Similarly, when people multitask while exercising, they might be taxing their brains.

[11]For example, the average American supermarket carries about 30,000 different unique items, increasing the number of decisions people must make.

coping with loneliness suffer impaired self-control and clear thinking. They struggle to make themselves feel better, if only for the moment.[12]

Age

Early in life, the reflective system is poorly developed and willpower is relatively weak. Children's behavior is more dominated by the affective system. They tend to behave in a manner in which they feel like doing whatever they want right now, without much thought about the future. However, as they age, they learn to constrain many desires and behaviors that conflict with social rules and that lead to negative consequences. This is the first sign of the development of willpower and an example of how the reflective system gains control over the emotion system.

Blood Sugar

Some have suggested that blood sugar, which brain cells use as their main energy source and cannot do without for even a few minutes, has an impact upon our willpower (Gailliot et al., 2007). Most cognitive functions are unaffected by minor blood sugar fluctuations over the course of a day, but willpower strength is sensitive to such small changes. Exerting willpower lowers blood sugar, which reduces the capacity for further self-control. Research shows that people who drink a glass of lemonade between completing tasks that required self-control performed equally well on both tasks. However, drinking sugarless diet lemonade was not as effective (Gailliot & Baumeister, 2007). Dieting essentially involves restricting one's caloric intake and produces lower glucose, which, in turn, undermines the willpower needed to refrain from eating. Foods that persistently elevate blood sugar, such as those containing protein or complex carbohydrates, might enhance willpower for longer periods.

Willpower as Mental Muscle

The good news, however, is that practice increases willpower capacity. Like a muscle, willpower seems to become stronger with use. However, willpower decreases as a result of its nonuse. For example, people living

---

[12]There is also evidence that women's menstrual cycles deplete willpower. Karen Pine and Ben Fletcher (2011) report that women in their cycle have lower self-regulatory resources and tend to make "impulsive purchases."

in a society with a limited choice set may become increasingly unable to effectively exercise self-control (Elster, 2006). Self-control theorists have suggested that willpower strength can be cultivated—just as muscular strength can be developed—so that repeated exercises of self-control in one domain (such as dieting) may make future displays of self-control easier, both in the domain of dieting and in other domains. Loewenstein, Read, and Baumeister (2003) suggest that sleep may be one way that individuals can replenish self-control. Most forms of self-regulation failure escalate over the course of the day, becoming more likely and more frequent the longer the person has been deprived of sleep. Positive emotional experience may also help replace expended self-control energy. Evidence shows that positive emotions can recharge a depleted self-regulatory system (Tice, Baumeister, Shmueli, & Muraven, 2007). The idea of exercising willpower is seen in military boot camp, where recruits are trained to overcome one challenge after another.

Autonomous Self-Control

Exerting self-control for personal reasons is less depleting. Decisions that feel autonomous (personally chosen) lead to less depletion and better self-control performance than making forced choices. People with an intrinsic motivation do not have to use their limited capacity of willpower. For example, people who diet for more personal reasons tend to be more successful at losing weight than people who diet for external reasons (Muraven, 2008). Autonomous self-control may involve less feelings of internal conflict and may be more energizing.[13] Thus, exerting self-control for personal reasons is less depleting. Also making choice that fits one's own preferences is less depleting. In short, enjoyable decisions are less depleting.

How to Balance the "Willpower Budget"

The allocation of willpower is an important decision that people face. In the short term, you should spend your limited "willpower budget" wisely. For example, it can be counterproductive to work toward multiple goals at the same time if your willpower cannot cover all the efforts that are required. Concentrating your effort on one or at most a few goals at a time increases the odds of success. For example, it makes no sense

---

[13]In general, when you feel passionate about your goal, you behave passively rather than making efforts to initiate your action.

to "decide" that one is going to quit smoking and diet if one does not actually allocate (or possess) the requisite willpower to actually follow through with both resolutions.

ERRONEOUS SENSE-MAKING

We have far more introspective access to cognitive than to emotional processes. Consequently, we tend to interpret our own behavior as a result of deliberate decision making even when this is not the case (Wilson, 2002). We tend to quickly come up with explanations for things we do not really have an explanation for. The reasons that people give when asked to explain their own behavior are rarely insightful—they are generally rationalizations. Humans are prone to retrospective justifications. We feel pressed to understand and to justify our emotions, and we retrospectively justify our action (Wilson, 2002). For example, the person who has consumed the tempting good but feels guilty about it may try to alleviate his guilt. He would do so by coming up with additional reasons that justify his behavior.

It is a fundamental feature of human beings that they have an image of themselves as acting for a reason. Ramachandran (2004) remarks that our conscious life is nothing but an elaborate post hoc[14] rationalization of things that we really do for other reasons. Robert Wright (1994) points out that the brain is like a good lawyer and, like a lawyer, the human brain wants victory, not truth. Michael Gazzaniga (2008) argues that the pressure to justify one's actions reflects the operation of "an interpreter system" housed in the left-hemisphere brain. The interpreter is driven to generate explanations and hypotheses regardless of circumstances. The left hemisphere may generate a feeling in all of us that we are integrated and unified. Gazzaniga claims that the interpreter is behind the human adoration of reason. People engage in confabulation—they readily fabricate reasons to explain their own behavior. In short, the brain does not necessarily seek to obtain "objective" truth about the world. It assigns itself a goal and assesses reality with respect to the goal. In other words, the brain only perceives what it wishes to. Thus, making sense is a deep human motivator, but making sense is not the same as being correct.

Wilson (2002) reports a number of carefully structured experimental situations in which people were required to do things and then say why they did what they did. In one study, they lined up several pairs of stockings on a table. Female subjects were then allowed to examine the

---

[14]Post hoc fallacy is a logical error that simply because one thing occurs after another, the first event is concluded to be a cause of the second one.

stockings and to choose which one they liked best. When the women were questioned, they had all sorts of wonderful answers about the texture and sheerness of the stockings that justified their choices. But unbeknownst to them, the stockings were identical. The subjects believed that they had decided on the basis of their internal judgments about the quality of the stockings.

In another experiment, an investigator (Wilson & Gilbert, 2005) had students in a photography class at Harvard choose two favorite pictures from among those they had just taken and then relinquish one to the teacher. Some students were told their choices were permanent; others were told they could exchange their prints after several days. As it turned out, those who had time to change their minds were less pleased with their decisions than those whose choices were irrevocable. Why did introspection interfere with their reactions? Wilson argues that "thinking too much" about the picture caused the subjects to focus on all sorts of variables that did not actually matter.[15] Instead of just listening to their affective preferences, their rational brains searched for reasons to prefer one picture for another. When we overanalyze, we ignore the wisdom of our emotions, which are much better in assessing our preferences.[16] A major implication of the mind's tendency for erroneous sense-making is that one needs to be suspicious to view one's own behavior as the outcome of deliberations.[17] Introspective understanding of the causes of emotion states can be limited, especially when people are asked to reflect back on an episode after it is over. Emotions are difficult to verbalize.[18]

CONCLUSION

This chapter has demonstrated that individual behavior is best understood as the outcome of a struggle between an emotion system and a reflective system. These two systems use different modes of operations that lead to different behavior. The final choice will depend on the relative

---

[15]In one experiment, a white rat in a maze repeatedly beat groups of Yale undergraduates in understanding the optimal way to get food dropped in the maze. The students overanalyzed and saw patterns that did not exist, so they were beaten by the rodent.

[16]This experiment also challenges our common assumption that we would be happier with the option to change our minds when in fact we are happier with closure.

[17]Donald Hebb once noted that outside observers are far more accurate at judging a person's true emotional state than is the person himself.

[18]Some economists argue that free market does not automatically produce what people really want. Rather, it produces what they *think* they want and are willing to pay for. If consumers are willing to pay for snake oil, the market will produce snake oil (Akerlof & Shiller, 2009).

strength of the competing systems. For example, under conditions of sufficient available self-control resources, the deliberative system will have the upper hand. However, under conditions of cognitive load, the reflective system may fail to activate inhibitory action. Consequently, impulses should better predict choices. The key insight here is that, rather than thinking about our decision as being governed by a unitary preference, it can often be better described in terms of the interaction between different subsystems that might favor different alternatives for a given decision. Maintaining a healthy balance between the affective system and the deliberative system remains one of the fundamental challenges of human beings.

The understanding of the role of emotion in decision making helps to recognize that people's food choices involve both automatic and reflective processes. This approach integrates each of two systems as well as environmental conditions in behavior determination. The framework provides a more realistic explanation of unhealthy behaviors. The intervention strategies to promote healthy behavior that rely primarily on health messages (reflective process) will have limited impact on behavior change. A more effective approach will address both automatic processes and reflective determinants of health behavior. For example, impulse-oriented interventions may target tempting stimuli triggered by situational cues that lead to excessive consumption. Thus, paying attention to the affective determinants of eating behavior complements the traditional approach intended to improve deliberative system, such as changing attitudes and beliefs.

8

Food Addiction and Obesity

INTRODUCTION

Recent studies (Volkow & Wise, 2005) show the similarity between overeating and addictive behaviors. The purpose of this chapter is to describe the similarity between overeating and addictive behaviors. The concept of addiction provides insight into why some obese individuals continue to struggle to change their food behaviors. The conceptualization of overeating as addiction informs understanding of the psychological factors that contribute to overeating and a useful framework for designing effective prevention and treatment programs.[1]

OVEREATING AS AN ADDICTIVE BEHAVIOR

Overeating exists despite an awareness of its poor health outcomes. With widespread warnings from the medical and public health community, it is safe to assume that people are generally informed about the negative consequences of poor nutrition and obesity. Moreover, efforts to reduce weight have been resistant to known treatment approaches. In spite of billions of dollars spent on weight loss[2] products, there has not been any successful solution. The addiction framework may provide an explanation for the irrational[3] overeating.

There is a body of research that shows that processed foods with high concentrations of sugar and fats are addictive, and many people lose control over their ability to regulate their consumption of such foods (Volkow & Wise, 2005). The addictive quality of these foods[4] could account for the

---

[1]While media may seem to glamorize drug addiction, food addicts can experience the opposite effect. Food also differs from other addictive substances because it is legal and relatively cheap.
[2]The limited success of weight loss programs may be due to the incomplete understanding of the factors that increase the risk of obesity.
[3]People knowingly engage in self-defeating behavior.
[4]Foods frequently involved in overeating episodes include pizza, hamburgers, cookies, chips, and desserts.

prevalence of obesity. The mechanisms through which these foods lead to excessive food consumption are likely to involve reward systems in the brain (e.g., dopamine and opiate systems) that create powerful motivations to eat. Consumption of highly palatable foods can enhance mood in a manner similar to other addictive substances. Adults with binge eating disorders (BED) show enhanced preference for sweet and fatty foods compared with other obese individuals (Davis et al., 2007).

The food industry has become especially savvy in exploiting our natural desire for sugar and fat by adding more of these ingredients in much of our daily foods. For example, between 1970 and 2000, there was a 42% per capita increase in the consumption of added fats and a 162% increase in cheese relative to only a 20% increase in fruits and vegetables (U.S. Department of Agriculture [USDA], 2010). The same study reported that per capita soft-drink consumption has increased by almost 500% in the past 50 years. The sharply reduced cost of sugar and vegetable oils worldwide has greatly contributed to the production of highly palatable processed foods (Drewnowski & Darmon, 2005). The annual growth rate of "fast food" dining has increased three-fold in the past generation, compared with that of at-home consumption (Currie, Vigna, Moretti, & Pathania, 2009). Fast foods are inherently addictive because of their concentration and high volume of fats and sugars.

Evolutionary biologists believe that the motivation to ingest foods high in energy density (sugar and fat) evolved to enhance human energy intake in unpredictable nutritional environments.[5] The desire for energy-dense foods had a strong survival advantage. Because the majority of surplus energy is stored as fat, this would help ensure survival during intermittent periods of food scarcity. However, in the quantities that many people consume them today, they have an abuse potential rivaling popular addictive drugs.

DEFINING ADDICTION

Addiction is defined as compulsive drug use despite negative consequences (Koob, 2003). Addiction begins with some experimentation and pleasurable responses. For subgroups of individuals, the initial use is followed by preoccupation, escalation, tolerance, and what has been referred to as a "fatal attraction" between the substance (or activity, for example, gambling) and the user (Elster, 1999). Obviously, the process resulting

---

[5]As noted before, preference for sweet is shown to be present in infants and exists independently of familiarity or learning.

in addiction is not fulfilled in all or even most users.[6] The *Diagnostic and Statistical Manual for Mental Disorders (DSM-IV)* defines substance dependence when three or more of the seven criteria listed below occur within 1 year. This section illustrates food consumption in a manner consistent with the seven diagnostic criteria of addictive behavior (Gearhardt, Corbin, & Brownell, 2009).

DSM-IV substance dependence criteria:

1. Tolerance
2. Withdrawal symptoms
3. Substance taken in larger amounts and for longer periods than intended
4. Persistent desire or repeated attempts to quit
5. Excessive time spent to obtain, use, or recover from use
6. Important social, occupational, or recreational activities given up or reduced
7. Continue to use despite knowledge of adverse consequences

Loss of Control

Loss of control is indicated by the frequent consumption of a substance in greater amounts or over longer periods of time than was initially intended. Loss of control is perhaps the most obvious feature of addictive behavior, even in the face of detrimental consequences to health, safety, social relationships, and financial stability. Loss of control is a part of a diagnosis in patients with BED and bulimia nervosa (BN).

Binging is a first stage of addiction. Binging[7] is defined as the escalation of intake with a high proportion of intake at one time, usually after a period of voluntary abstinence. Binge eating is often accompanied by feelings of loss of control and psychological distress. Individuals engaging in binge eating will eat until they feel uncomfortably full and may or may not compensate for the overeating. Binges can be triggered by the consumption of a "forbidden food" that is often high in fat and/or

---

[6]There are a number of host or individual factors, such as genetics, intrauterine exposure, early childhood, and adolescence experience, that influence susceptibility and/or resilience.

[7]Binge episodes are associated with at least three of the following criteria: (1) eating more rapidly than normal, (2) eating when not physically hungry, (3) eating until uncomfortably full, (4) eating alone because of shame, and (5) feeling disgusted with oneself, depressed, or guilty after overeating.

sugar, followed by uncontrolled consumption of food in quantities as high as 5,000 calories (Ifland et al., 2009).

Adults suffering from BED tend to describe themselves as "food addicts" or "compulsive overeaters" (Cassin & von Ranson, 2007). They typically report distress and guilt about their eating habits and have great difficulty controlling these behaviors, despite unhealthy weight gain and ensuing medical problems, such as diabetes and hypertension.

Overweight and obesity are normally associated with binge eating. Approximately 9% of normal weight and 21% of overweight women report occasionally binge eating (Gearhardt et al., 2009). Thus, the existence of a loss of control over food consumption for a substantial proportion of the population is well documented (Gearhardt et al., 2009).

Tolerance

Tolerance occurs when one needs to consume greater quantities of a substance to achieve a desired effect or the substance has a diminished effect after continued use. Some behavioral evidence shows the development of food tolerance in patients with BN. Brown, Spanos, and Devlin (2007) found that as illness duration increases, binges become more frequent and the quantity of food consumed during binges increases.

High-fat/-sugar foods are initially ingested by most people during infancy or early childhood. Research suggests that there is a possibility that tolerance may develop during the early years. For example, Harrison (2008) found that sucrose is an effective analgesic for minor pains in young infants (similar to traditional opiates), but this effect is no longer evident after 18 months of age when many children have already begun to regularly consume high-sugar foods.

Withdrawal

The impact of tolerance on the progression of addictive behaviors is revealed by the debilitating symptoms of *withdrawal*. Withdrawal is defined as the development of physiological or cognitive symptoms in response to periods of abstinence or reduced consumption of a substance. Withdrawal can also be indicated by the consumption of a substance to prevent these symptoms from arising. Early-morning headache is the first sign of caffeine withdrawal, and caffeine addicts know how to cure it with that first morning cup of coffee. Certain foods (e.g., sweets) can cause pronounced withdrawal symptoms when removed from the diet. For instance, when either obese or lean humans restrict their food consumption, physiological responses are exaggerated, which reflect low blood sugar. The low level of sugar in the blood is associated with discomfort or fainting, as well as intense cravings and hunger (Hoebel, Avena, & Rada, 2007). This process is similar to the development of withdrawal in addicts, for whom anticipatory responses to drug cues result in physiologic changes that trigger cravings and sometimes relapse.

Cravings

One of the most distinguishing features of drug abuse is the pronounced sense of craving (or urge) reported by addicts and their dismal and repeated failures at giving up the habit. Craving is a subjective feeling of a strong urge to do something. Food craving[8] is defined as an irresistible urge to consume a specific food, strong enough that you may go out of your way to get it. Of central importance to the manifestation of craving is the obstacle to consumption. The individual will not experience craving if she or he responds in an automatic manner without cognitive effort to consume his or her favorite food. Craving occurs because he or she wishes to remain abstinent. Just knowing you cannot have a certain food could make you crave it. After all, forbidden fruit is more tempting. Studies have demonstrated that food cravings are significantly higher in adults with BED than in their non-binging counterparts of comparable weight (Cassin & von Ranson, 2007).

Food cravings, however, are not always pathological. Cravings are also triggered by nutritional deficiency. Food cravings are a means of ensuring a varied diet.[9] Many monotonous diets are nutritionally unbalanced, so cravings might be the body's way of encouraging you to eat a more varied diet.

Relapse

The addict's powerful cravings that can be elicited from even a small "dose," as well as from the many conditioned environmental cues, are thought to contribute to poor long-term treatment outcome. Leshner (1997)

---

[8]Chocolate is the food most typically associated with reports of food craving, although other energy-dense foods, including cakes, biscuits, and various salty and savory "snack" foods, also usually appear high on lists of craved foods. There is a difference between hunger and a craving. Hunger can be satisfied by eating any kind of food, whereas a craving can usually only be satisfied with a specific type of food. For example, a craving for pizza cannot be satisfied with spaghetti in tomato sauce. Oftentimes, not just any pizza will do. People will go out of their way to buy a particular brand or type of pizza.

[9]For example, cravings for chocolate may be influenced by a deficiency in magnesium; this may be why some experience an increase in chocolate cravings during PMS.

coined the term "chronic relapsing disorder" to describe these disorders because total and permanent abstinence seldom occurs after a single treatment episode. For most individuals, there are repeated cycles of quit and relapse. Human weight cycling is, almost by definition, a sign of repeated defeat in one's effort to curb overeating and is found to be a significant risk factor for binge eating (Petroni et al., 2007).

Continued Use Despite Physical or Psychological Harm

The association of high-calorie consumption and obesity with a host of serious health problems, such as heart disease and diabetes, provides some indication of continued use despite dire consequences.

A Desire to Reduce or Stop Consumption

The desire to reduce or quit consuming certain foods is pervasive in our society.[10] Dieting is frequently directed at abstaining from certain types of food and restricting overeating. The repeated failure of such attempts is evident in one study, in which 83% of participants regained their lost weight within 5 years (Davis et al., 2007). Presumably, these people did not plan to overeat and regain the weight.

A Great Deal of Time Spent in Activities Necessary to Obtain, Use, or Recover

Patients with BN or BED spend a great deal of time dealing with the emotional consequences of excess food consumption, including physical and psychological stress. In addition, dieters spend a great deal of time buying diet foods, being concerned with their weight, and so on.

Giving Up Other Important Activities

Being overweight is associated with decreased involvement in important life activities. Excessive food consumption and obesity may lead to low rates of physical activity and less engagement in social activities[11] (such

---

[10]Schwartz, Vartanian, Nosek, and Brownell (2006) studied 4,283 individuals and found that 46% would give up a year of their life instead of being obese; 15% would give up 10 years of life; 30% would rather be divorced; 25% would rather not be able to have children; and 14% would rather be alcoholic.
[11]This may be due in part to the experience of weight bias.

as dating or marriage) (Ifland et al., 2009). The drive to consume palatable foods may become so appealing that eating is frequently chosen over other important activities.

Summary

This section showed that elements of the addiction can be applied to food consumption in a manner consistent with the seven diagnostic criteria of addictive behavior.

Applying DSM-IV criteria to foods (Ifland et al., 2009), food addiction is defined when three or more of the seven criteria are occurring within 1 year.

1. **Tolerance:** Have you found that you need to eat a lot more than you used to in order to get the feeling you want?
2. **Withdrawal:** Do you eat to alleviate the feelings of depression, tiredness, anxiety, and agitation?
3. **Use more than intended:** Have you often found that when you started eating you ended up eating more than you originally intended?
4. **Tried to cut back:** Have you tried to cut down or stop overeating foods? Is this something you keep worrying about?
5. **Spend time pursuing, using, or recovering from use:** Have you spent a lot of time feeling uncomfortable or tired from eating?
6. **Missed important activities:** Have you had times when you would eat instead of working or spending time at hobbies or with family or friends?
7. **Eating in spite of knowledge of consequences:** Has your eating caused any psychological problems, such as making you depressed or anxious, making it difficult to sleep, or causing disruptive fatigue/physical problems?

SUGAR ADDICTION

The most common targets of food cravings and addictions are energy-dense foods that are sweet, high in fat, or both. Research on food addiction has thus far has focused on one macronutrient, sugar.[12] The most compelling evidence comes from animal studies showing that under some circumstances, sweet foods can be addictive. For example, Bart Hoebel (1999) has shown that rats binging on sugar release dopamine in the same way as rats given high doses of addictive drugs, and doing

---

[12]Although more data are needed, salt has been proposed to produce dependence (Cocores & Gold, 2009). Salted foods stimulate opiates and dopamine in the brain reward system. Salted food stimulates appetite and increases overeating.

so can cause lasting changes in the dopamine system, withdrawal symp-tom, and cross-sensitization to other drugs, including amphetamines. He argues that very sweet foods can induce a form of dependency.

Avena et al. (2008) have shown that a prolonged cycle of binge feeding on sugar foods may foster addiction. The experiment involved placing rats on a cycle of no food for 12 hours, followed by 12 hours of regular food plus a sugar solution (a 25% glucose solution). Hence, the rats were binge feeding on sugar for alternating 12-hour spans. As time progressed, the rats consumed an increasing amount of the sugar solu-tion. After about 3 weeks, the rats experienced an increase in brain recep-tors for opiates and dopamine.[13]

In sum, the research on animal studies shows that a cycle of depriva-tion and excessive sugar intake reinforces binging. Abstinence also trig-gers withdrawal symptoms that resemble those of drug addiction, such as anxiety, chattering teeth, and tremors. Following its removal, they show aggression, anxiety, a drop in body temperature, teeth chattering, forepaw tremor, and headshaking—all symptoms associated with with-drawal from drugs such as heroin. Furthermore, these studies suggest that the way in which food is used (going on and off diets) rather than its palatability may produce the food addiction.

For humans, the evidence suggests that that sugar may be addictive for some individuals when consumed in a "binge-like" manner and that sugar binging can cause lasting changes in the brain, in that sensitization remains after a period of normal feeding. Many people claim that they feel compelled to eat sweet foods, similar in some ways to how an alco-holic might feel compelled to drink. In these accounts, people describe symptoms of withdrawal when they deprive themselves of sugar-rich foods. Anecdotal information on human "sugar withdrawal" consists of headaches and irritability among heavy sugar consumers who become abstinent. They also describe food cravings, particularly for sugar and other carbohydrates, which can trigger impulsive eating. For example, in his low carbohydrate diet book (Atkins, 2002), Atkins warned that an abrupt decline in carbohydrates could provoke "fatigue, faintness, palpitations, headaches, and cold sweats."

EATING DISORDERS

Traditionally, food addiction has been treated as an "eating disorder" in the DSM. Eating disorders are an important and growing health concern

---

[13]Opiates are chemical messengers that identify sweet tastes as desirable, whereas dopa-mine is a chemical messenger that works with memory to urge people to pursue sweet tastes in the future.

in the United States. They hijack the natural eating process. The human body is designed to eat, and eating stops under normal circumstances only when the body senses it has enough energy for its immediate needs and enough stored away for future tasks.

The three officially recognized eating disorders are anorexia nervosa (AN), BN, and BED. AN and BN are frequently chronic and often disabling conditions that are characterized by abnormal patterns of eating behavior, and deviant attitudes and perceptions toward body weight and shape. Individuals with AN and BN have elevated rates of lifetime diagnoses of anxiety and depressive disorders, and obsessive-compulsive disorder. People with both disorders tend to organize their days around eating and allow food to loom too large in their lives. Food for them is much more than a source of nourishment; it can become a substitute for self-esteem and a vehicle for exercising, or losing, control over the body. Furthermore, only about half of the patients diagnosed with BN fully recover, many experiencing bulimic episodes for decades (Keel et al., 2005).

According to the National Institute of Mental Health (2006), an estimated 0.5% to 3.7% of women develop AN and some 1.1% to 4.2% experience BN in their lifetime. The incidence and prevalence of eating disorders in males is much lower—approximately 5% to 10% of the rate in females. Overall, the National Eating Disorders Association (National Eating Disorders Association [NEDA], 2008) reports that approximately 9 million women in the United States struggle with an eating disorder (ED).[14] BN accounts for the highest number of ED incidents and disproportionately affects women.

Approximately 8.4% of female adolescents reported purging to lose weight (National Youth Risk Behavior Survey, 2005). Among teens (9 to 15), females were more likely to start purging than binging, and males were more inclined to binge than to purge, and this all had to do with the teens' basic insecurities (National Youth Risk Behavior Survey, 2005). For males, the strongest predictors of binging were concern about their weight and negative comments about their weight by their fathers. Females under 14 whose mothers had histories of disordered eating were three times more likely than the others to start purging.

Mothers of girls with eating disorders may well have an influence on their daughters' pathology. In fact, 50% of children of mothers with eating disorders have psychiatric disorders (Alison et al., 2008). Twin and family studies suggest that AN, BN, and BED are complex genetic diseases, and for each disorder the estimated heritability ranges between 50% and 83% (Hudson & Pope, 2007). Thus, the occurrence of eating and

---

[14]To put this in perspective, in 2005, approximately 4.5 million people had Alzheimer disease and about 2.2 million had schizophrenia.

personality disturbance may be at least partly attributed to family interaction patterns, both neurobiological (e.g., serotonin levels) and hereditary (Cassin & Ranson, 2007).

Anorexia Nervosa

People suffering from AN starve themselves, exercise excessively, and still think they are too fat. Through sheer force of will, anorexics convince their body that it does not need food. Their extreme behavior is often driven by an inappropriate and distorted body image.[15] The result includes excessive weight loss and malnutrition, as well as symptoms of low blood pressure, slow heartbeat, constipation, osteoporosis, weakened immunity, and failure to menstruate. Treatment is often difficult, and death occurs in about 6% of cases (Alison et al., 2008). At least two thirds of anorexics do not fully recover even after years of the current treatment (Alison et al., 2008).

Most people greatly dislike dieting. But a person with AN actually feels better—more alert and energetic. They do not feel hunger pangs; they simply find ways to override them. Dieting becomes the ultimate accomplishment, a fix that the person with AN learns to crave (addiction to starvation). They also derive emotional gratification by avoiding food and achieving slimness (albeit never enough). The illness is accompanied by disturbances in the brain's reward system that may lead to a general inability to feel delight from life's pleasures (e.g., food, sex, or winning a lottery). People with anorexia have difficulty living in the here and now. They tend to live in the future, planning for all contingencies, and to largely disregard the present. Individuals with AN are more likely to have personality traits[16] of perfectionism, marked rigidity, conformity, narcissism, and reduced social spontaneity (Kaye, 2008). They have enhanced ability to pay attention to detail or use a logical/analytic approach but exhibit worse performance with global thinking. They also suffer from chronic anxiety (80% to 90%) (Kaye, 2008).

---

[15]A female is considered at risk if she is trying to lose weight and weighs less than 85% of the minimum normal weight for her height. This corresponds to a BMI range of 17.1–18.9 for young females ages 15–29.

[16]Evidence (Cassin & Ranson, 2007) shows that personality traits are associated with eating disorders. The individual uses the inappropriate behavior to exert control over her life. For example, the narcissist's pathological concern with appearance, intense interpersonal sensitivity, and need for validation from the external environment create vulnerability for eating disorders. Similarly, perfectionism is characterized by the tendency to set and pursue unrealistically high standard, despite the adverse consequences. The literature suggests that personality should be considered in the diagnosis of eating disorders. In particular, impulsivity precedes the development of bulimia.

Poor nutrition has a general effect on brain function. The brain is particularly vulnerable to the consequences of poor nutrition since it uses around 20% of the caloric intake and is especially dependent on glucose (Sodersten, Bergh, & Zandian, 2006). Since most eating disorders emerge during adolescence (a vulnerable period of brain reorganization), malnutrition during this crucial period is associated with impaired judgment. Many symptoms resolve with weight gain and when brain mass is restored. So, starvation/eating disorder leads to the impaired judgment and psychiatric symptoms associated with AN (Sodersten et al., 2006). Thus, it is important to correct these false beliefs regarding body image, the fattening effects of certain foods, and so forth. This suggests that the timing of information provision may be crucial. Getting information about risks to the potential anorexic before impaired judgment sets in may have a much higher payoff than the information that arrives after the judgment becomes impaired. Changes in broader societal attitudes about the attractiveness of extreme thinness would also counteract tendencies to anorexia.[17]

Bulimia Nervosa

Bulimics often restrict intake early in the day and then binge later in the evening usually on palatable foods. Typically, extremely large amounts of food (> 3,000 kcal) are consumed during bulimic episodes, with most items being palatable (energy-dense, high-fat, high-carbohydrate foods) (Kaye, 2008). Bulimics struggle to control their binges and are forced to engage in purging (most notably in the form of vomiting, but also through laxatives and strenuous exercise). Bulimia is often called the "invisible" eating disorder because you cannot tell by looking at someone's body that she or he has it. There are serious health consequences from these binge and purge cycles, including electrolyte imbalances that can cause irregular heartbeats, heart failure, inflammation and possible rupture of the esophagus from frequent vomiting, tooth decay, gastric rupture, muscle weakness, anemia, and malnutrition (American Psychiatric Association, 1993).

---

[17]A similar condition to anorexia is known as orthorexia. It is included under the catch-all label EDNOS. The condition was named by a Californian doctor, Steven Bratman, in 1997 and is described as a "fixation on righteous eating." The condition affects equal numbers of men and women aged over 30, middle-class, and well-educated. Their dietary restrictions commonly cause sufferers to feel proud of their "virtuous" behavior even if it means that eating becomes so stressful their personal relationships can come under pressure and they become socially isolated. They feel incredibly guilty if they eat something that they consider unhealthy. They are critical about what other people eat. Eating only healthy food gives them a sense of control about their life, particularly when everything else seems out of control.

Binge eating in bulimic subjects might be understood as the undesired outcome of restrained eating and obesity prevention. In most cases, bulimia develops several months after the onset of dieting (Kaye, 2008). Some 25% to 30% of bulimics have a prior history of AN (Kaye, 2008). Chronic dieters restrain their food intake until a disinhibitor causes a temporary break in the diet regimen with overeating.

Similar to addiction, binge eating is a form of self-defeating behavior that normally occurs amid attempts to lose weight by restricting one's caloric intake. Binge eating also alters mood, perhaps mainly by providing escape from distress. Finally, a variety of physiological adaptations are likely to be important in the binge eater's capacity to tolerate very large meals (Rogers & Smit, 2000).

Individuals with BN are more likely to have high impulsivity and engage in sensation-seeking and novelty-seeking behaviors (Davis et al., 2007). Sexual promiscuity, suicide attempts, drug abuse, and stealing or shoplifting are frequently noted in these patients (Kaye, 2008).

The study of BN presents several important policy implications. First, since addiction is the most important cause of BN persistence, it is reasonable to expect that the longer an individual experiences BN the less responsive she will be to treatment. In this respect it is important to instruct a wide range of young women on the deleterious effects of BN and the importance of getting help, especially at the initial stages of bulimic behaviors. Second, BN should be treated as an addiction, rather than only as a disorder. This change would put those exhibiting BN on equal footing (from a treatment reimbursement perspective) with individuals abusing drugs or alcohol.

Binge Eating Disorder

Bing eating disorder is currently classified in the "eating disorders not otherwise specified" (EDNOS) category.[18] Binge eating afflicts approximately 5% of U.S. adults at some time in their lives (Corwin & Grigson, 2009). Binge eating constitutes a significant public health concern by virtue of its strong associations with other medical and psychiatric disorders, most notably obesity and depression (Corwin & Grigson, 2009).

Binge eating is characterized by discrete episodes of rapid and excessive food consumption not necessarily driven by hunger or metabolic

---

[18]Also included in this category is probable BN (PBN), which is defined in terms of binge eating episodes and compensatory behaviors that occur less than twice a week or for a duration of less than 3 months. PBN was found to be more common in a large sample of college students (20%–30%) than BN that meets full criteria.

need. BED differs from BN in that binging is not followed by vomiting, the use of laxatives, or excessive exercise. Binge eating is often accompanied by feelings of loss of control and psychological distress. Not surprisingly, overweight and obesity are commonly accompanied with binge eating.

As noted before, animal studies show that putting animals through repeated cycles of food deprivation followed by exposure to palatable food leads to overeating. This is similar to someone who goes on a strict diet, then goes off the wagon with a palatable meal, again and again over a period of time. This repeated pattern leads to binge eating. The behavior also leads to changes in reward system in the brain. Researchers have concluded that "even highly palatable food is not addictive in and of itself. Rather, it is the manner in which the food is presented (i.e., intermittently) and consumed (i.e., repeated, intermittent "gorging") that appears to entrain the addiction-like process" (Corwin & Grigson, 2009).

The American Psychiatric Association offers a number of criteria for BED (American Psychiatric Association [APA], 2000). Three or more of the following are associated with the binge-eating episodes. These behaviors occur at least twice a week for 6 months:

1. Eating a larger amount of food than normal during a short period of time (within any 2-hour period)
2. Eating until feeling uncomfortably full, to the point of discomfort
3. Eating large amounts of food when not physically hungry
4. Eating alone because the person is embarrassed by the amount of food consumed
5. Feeling disgusted, depressed, or guilty after overeating

The majority of BED patients meet the criteria for binge-eating addiction. Evidence shows that binge eating, like addiction, involves the endogenous opioid system and the dopamine system. The opioid system is involved with the liking and the pleasurable responses to food that reinforces the intake of highly palatable foods, such as those consumed in a high-fat and high-sugar diet. As will be discussed in the next chapter, low levels of dopamine D_2 receptors have been reported in individuals with eating disorders. Thus, compulsive overeating may occur to compensate for reduced activation of the dopamine system, which may predispose these patients to seek food as a means to self-medicate. Decreased dopamine levels are also associated with decreased activity in prefrontal regions involved in inhibitory control, which may underlie their inability to control food intake. A recent survey found that as many as 42.3% of clinicians tend to use addiction-based treatment for BED patients (von Ranson & Robinson, 2006).

Summary

For all their differences, anorexia, bulimia, and binge eating exist along a continuum and usually emerge after a period of dieting. Those who succumb typically start out hoping to lose a few pounds but end up obsessing about food/eating and weight/shape. But frequent and extreme dieting quickly disturbs the body's hunger-satiety system, leading to eating disorder and faulty perception.

Stress eating is a huge issue and tops the list of triggers for eating disorders. Emotional stress shift priorities to the immediate present. Eating reduces stress or anxiety by increasing feelings of pleasure derived from consuming palatable foods. However, the effect is usually short-lived and followed by shame, guilt, or other negative feelings. Thus, life events create stressful events for which binge eating becomes the solution. That is, eating disorder is a symptom and not the cause of the problem. Instead of dealing with the stress, the binge eater uses food as a strategy to regulate negative emotion. By focusing one's attention onto weight, shape, and eating, one enters a domain in which one can gain some emotional control. The obsessive focus on weight loss and its associated tactics provides a narrow, apparently viable way to avoid dealing with broader issues (Herman & Polivy, 2002).

THE POWER OF HABIT

It is important to note that not all cases of excessive food consumption are viewed as addictive behavior. For some individuals, overeating is a relatively mindless behavior, in the form of frequent snacking and large portion sizes. For others, as noted above, it can be compulsive and excessively driven.

Habits are learned slowly, but once they are in place, they are inflexible and difficult to break.[19] The term habit refers to any activity that involves a significant element of automaticity through associative learning (Wood & Neal, 2007, 2009). Once formed, the habitual response comes to be primed or triggered by the perception of cues, such as the physical setting in which the habit typically is performed. For example, when you come home, you head straight to the refrigerator. A habit is a way to save cognitive effort. However, the danger of habit for food is the loss of control.

---

[19]The English poet John Dryden (1631–1700) noted that "we first make our habits and then our habits make us."

Our preferences are strongly influenced by our past experiences. A history of personal experience gives particular foods an emotional charge, and those emotions become a part of our memory, which drive our behavior. Over time, the act of eating highly rewarding food creates an automatic response. The more we do it the behavior becomes habit-driven and less deliberate. As a result, our eating behavior becomes automatic. Habitual behaviors are triggered by specific cues or contexts. Cues in the environment become the triggers of predictable and automatic actions. The influence of habits on behavior is amplified by everyday demands (e.g., time pressures, distractions, and regulatory depletion) that limit the capacity to inhibit habitual response. As we repeatedly practice using a particular response to meet a goal, other alternative responses serving the same goal becomes less accessible in our memory.

Highly palatable foods have the capacity to rewire our brains, driving to seek more of those products. The actions that led to pleasure become imprinted on the brain and the habit of pursuit becomes firmly established. Our response becomes conditioned (when I am in this situation, I tend to act that way). Conditioned overeating overrides the executive control functions to restrict consuming highly palatable foods. Once we associate the eating behavior with a desired outcome, we begin to act more automatically to achieve that outcome.

Cues, priming, and emotions trigger conditioned overeating. Learned cues capture our attention and motivate us to act. By responding to a salient cue with action that generates immediate reward, we only strengthen the association between the cue and its reward. If you eat the salient food that you want today, it's going to be more salient tomorrow because you have more positive associations with it. Sometimes just one taste of a food is enough to prime conditioned overeating. Priming works in part by triggering memories of past pleasure and activating the pleasure centers of the brain. The power of priming is obvious in two highly palatable foods, pizza and ice cream. Finally, among people who experience conditioned overeating, emotional states often heighten the power of cues and intensify the urge to eat. It is a form of self-medication. People use the food to calm themselves down. Sadness and anger have the greatest potential to drive a loss of control. The beliefs that food makes us feel better contributes to our desire for food. Expecting something to be rewarding stimulates pursuit of that reward. The act of eating becomes something we do to attain a desired emotional effect. For example, because a cookie makes me feel better, it is easy to develop the habit of seeking it out when I am sad or angry. Over time, the association between mood and eating cookie grows stronger.

CONCLUSION

The theory of addition shares some aspects of the behavioral pattern in people diagnosed with eating disorders (such as binge eating disorder or bulimia). Similar to addicts, bulimics experience intense food cravings in response to food cues and stress. They learn that binge-eating alleviates anxiety, making them feel better at the time. After binging, bulimics frequently experience negative emotions, including guilt, self-disgust, fear of weight gain, and depression. In response, they engage in purging to reduce these negative emotional states. In the case of anorexia, it is argued that patients may be addicted to the release of endogenous opioids, which are released in self-starvation and excessive exercise. In short, starving, binging, purging, and exercise increase endorphin levels, resulting in the same chemical effect as that delivered by opiates.

This chapter outlined parallels between drug addiction in humans and compulsive overeating. This conceptualization of compulsive overeating can provide a helpful framework for developing more effective treatments for compulsive overeating. However, a major limitation for compulsive overeaters is the impossibility of completely abstaining from the "addictive substance" as is often recommended for drug addiction.[20] Framing compulsive overeating as an addiction presents BED patients with the implicit message that they may be fighting a strong neurobiological drive to overeat in an environment that exploits these urges. The model may help foster a therapeutic sense of self-empathy as well as an understanding that treatment is likely to involve learning effective strategies and enduring life-long efforts to resist overeating and prevent relapse.

Finally, it is important to note that the question whether food addiction leads to obesity remain unresolved. Overall, 11% of Americans suffer from an eating disorder (Benton, 2010). This number does not account for the 35% of the U.S. adult population that is overweight. Several factors are involved in obesity, and food addiction may be one of them.

---

[20]Some treatment approaches, such as Overeaters Anonymous, view compulsive overeating as a disease that sufferers are powerless to overcome and recommend "surrendering oneself to a higher power."

9

Overeating and Decision-Making Deficits

INTRODUCTION

The previous chapter discussed the similarity between overeating and addictive behavior. Similar to addictive behavior, some ingredients in palatable food (i.e., sweet, salty, and fat) activate brain circuitry that involves reward, motivation, decision making, learning, and memory. Factors that make people vulnerable to addiction also make them vulnerable to obesity. This chapter illustrates the role of brain reward system dysfunction in overeating and obesity. The chapter will demonstrate how dysfunction in decision making contributes to overeating and obesity. The result of dysfunction in decision making is an enhanced value of one type of reward (food for the obese individuals) at the expense of other rewards.

THE BRAIN'S PLEASURE CENTER

The brain's pleasure center evolved to foster our selective engagement in activities such as eating, sex, and social activities, which are the essence of our survival as a species. Evolution has designed us to enjoy things that are good for us. The attainment of a particular feeling is an important motive. For example, we are designed to have a taste for sweets. Individuals with a taste for the sugars would be more likely to have acquired the nutrients required for survival and reproduction. Loneliness prompts a desire to affiliate with others. Like hunger, it is a warning to do something to alter an uncomfortable and possibly dangerous condition.

The pleasure center is also at the heart of all addiction disorders. Abused substances activate the same brain reward pathways as life's natural pleasures. In other words, there is a shared substrate for food and drug reward. It is commonly suggested that drugs "hijack" the brain (enslave it to the pleasure of a particular substance). Addictive drugs not only reorganize the preference structure but also induce a dramatic change in the allocation of behavioral resources toward the addictive substance. Addicts will go to greater lengths to obtain their preferred drug, typically at the expense of other motivational activities. Addictive drugs do not serve any beneficial survival purpose, but instead often are harmful to health and well-being.

Reward and Motivation System

The vast majority of behavior is motivated by either obtaining rewards or avoiding punishment. A reward is defined as anything an animal will work for, whereas a punishment is anything an animal will work to avoid or escape. Reward is crucial to most human behavior. We do things that will bring rewarding outcomes or avoid outcomes that would be harmful or unpleasant. The motivation system is the system of forces that energize and direct our actions. The theory of addiction is in fact a theory of motivation and how the motivational system is distorted, in which a reward-seeking behavior has become out of control. This is an abnormally and damagingly high priority given to a particular activity.

Conditioned Learning

Conditioning is the process by which an originally neutral stimulus becomes associated with a primary reward, whereas *instrumental learning* is a process whereby animals learn to perform an action to obtain a reward or avoid a punishment. We learn which cues signal positive and negative outcomes and we learn how our actions and behaviors can increase the probability of positive outcomes. The process whereby behavior is modified by rewards and punishments is termed *reinforcement,* and a reinforcer is any stimulus that elicits behavioral modification. A *primary* (or *unconditioned*) *reinforcer* elicits motivated behavior without any learning. Examples of primary reinforcer include food and sex. These rewards do not need to be learned. A *secondary reinforcer* only elicits the response after learning has occurred. These rewards get their power by being paired with primary reinforcers.

Dopamine

Two of the major players in reward system are dopamine and the endogenous opiates. These pleasure chemicals provide ample evidence for similarity between food addiction and drug cravings.

Dopamine (a chemical central to the pleasure response) is an important regulator of food intake. Dopamine is released in anticipation of eating, which motivates us to search for and consume food. Dopamine is released again when food is consumed. People get a "dopamine rush" from eating chocolate or listening to music. Our engagement in these behaviors increases our sense of pleasure and well-being. Dopamine is about rewards and feeling good, and wanting to feel good again. We have the desire to repeat these behaviors even in the face of distracting stimuli.

The rewarding behaviors nurture a strong positive memory, which increases their salience and enhances our appetitive motivation to seek these behaviors. We quickly learn the cues in our environment, which signal the approach or availability of these rewarding behaviors. In the context of food intake, dopamine release may accompany the cues that anticipate eating, so that over time with repeated ingestion dopamine release shifts from food delivery (i.e., the pleasure of ingesting food) to cues associated with craving food (e.g., the sight and smell of food).

Dopamine plays an important role in understanding food addiction. For instance consider the case of weight gain after smoking cessation. Since nicotine and food stimulate the same dopamine reward circuitry, abstinent smokers may substitute food to stimulate the dopamine reward pathway. Similarly, there is an evidence of an inverse relation between alcohol consumption and body mass index (BMI) (Wang et al., 2001). The inverse relation is attributable to competition between food and alcohol for similar neurotransmitter receptors.[1] Alcohol and food use the same biological pathways, and when a pathway is occupied by one, it would block the other. When opiate blockers, such as naltrexone, are used to block reward pathways, binge eaters reduce their consumption of sweet high-fat foods, and alcohol-dependent participants reduce their consumption of alcohol (Gearhardt, Corbin, & Brownell, 2009). Thus, as BMI increases, alcohol consumption decreases. This inverse relationship is consistent with the theory that food may be addictive.

Other neurotransmitter systems, such as the opioids and serotonin, are also integral to the reward process. The opioids, also known as endorphins, are chemicals produced in the brain that have rewarding effects similar to drugs such as morphine and heroin. Consumption of high-sugar, high-fat foods can cause endogenous opiates to be released in the brain and relieve pain or stress and calm us down. It is also known that after using drugs that activate the opioid system, people report that palatable food is more pleasant, and they eat more of it. Using opiate blockers (block the production of opioids) such as naloxone can reduce the pleasure and craving for substances in addicts. Naloxone also reduces consumption and preference for sweet high-fat foods in both normal weight and obese binge eaters (Drewnowski & Darmon, 1995).

---

[1]An alternative explanation is the possibility that reduction in alcohol consumption may be due to negative social experiences. Since consumption of alcohol frequently takes place in social contexts, such as bars or parties, obese individuals due to discrimination reduce their participation in social activities in which alcohol consumption is common (Puhl & Brownell, 2001).

DISORDERS IN REWARD PROCESSING

As noted in earlier chapters, the prefrontal cortex (PFC) shares reciprocal connections with midbrain regions (e.g., the nucleus accumbens) that are important for reward. A universal feature of rewarding stimuli, such food or drugs of abuse, is that they activate dopamine release in the nucleus accumbens. This holds true even when obese persons view pictures of food items that lead to craving (Ifland et al., 2009). Addiction theory suggests that when the reward systems display an exaggerated sensitivity to drug cues, the reward systems are uncoupled from the PFC and addicts fail to control their consumption (Ifland et al., 2009). When the PFC becomes uncoupled from the reward system, the addict is no longer able to effectively regulate appetitive desires.

Theorists have posited that obesity results from abnormalities in reward processing (Stice, Yokum, Blum, & Bohon, 2010). Some researchers propose that a hyper-responsiveness of reward system to food intake increases the risk of overeating. The theory suggests that certain people show greater sensitivity of brain reward systems to food stimuli. The sensitivity of the reward system is affected in part by the brain's dopamine system. Individuals who are more reward-sensitive are more likely to detect rewarding stimuli and have a stronger drive to pursue behaviors with potentially pleasurable outcomes. For example, obese individuals rate high-fat and high-sugar foods as more pleasant and consume more of such foods than lean individuals. Preferences for high-fat and high-sugar foods predict elevated weight gain and increased risk of obesity (Davis et al., 2007).

Another view, known as *reward deficiency hypothesis*, argues that the reduced pleasure in some individuals causes them to eat more to attain a normal amount of pleasure (Volkow, Wang, Fowler, & Telang, 2008). It is hypothesized that deficits in D_2 receptors may predispose individuals to use psychoactive drugs or overeat to boost a sluggish dopamine reward system. The premise is that substances (such as addictive drugs and palatable food) are used as a form of "self-medication" to boost a sluggish dopamine system and increase hedonic capacity. Especially if they have previously experienced that binging has the capacity to alter a negative mood state in the short run, even though long-term consequences are potentially negative.[2] Researchers argue that overeating reflects a "reward

---

[2] According to the self-medication model of addiction, the addict may be taking drugs as a means of coping with or ameliorating adverse life experiences. For example, alcohol can help people to forget their troubles, calm fears, and ease pain. The model assumes that psychological problems precede drug use. For example, it is argued that individuals with particular problems with intimacy in personal relationships may have their needs met by an intense intimate relationship with a drug. This explains the observation that experience of abuse as a child predisposes to addiction to drugs such as alcohol and heroin.

deficiency" syndrome that could foster overeating as a compensatory behavior to increase dopamine receptor to a more comfortable level. Thus, obese individuals may experience less subjective reward from food intake because they have fewer D_2 receptors. Thus, high D_2 receptor levels could protect against drug self-administration.

Research shows that individuals with lower D_2 receptors had higher BMI. Imaging studies have shown that both obese individuals and drug-dependent individuals have significantly lower dopamine receptor levels[3] (Wang et al., 2001). Volkow et al. (2008) show that morbidly obese subjects (BMI > 40) had lower than normal D_2 receptors. Among adolescents, the lower dopamine response predicts future weight gain. These findings indicate that low D_2 receptor availability could be a risk factor for overeating. Consequently, in cultures where highly palatable foods are readily available, it is probable that these vulnerable individuals will eat more, and eat more often. Similarly, drug availability markedly increases the likelihood of drug abuse.

An alternative interpretation is that consumption of a high-fat, high-sugar diet leads to down-regulation of D_2 receptors (decreased sensitivity/dulling of the dopamine system), similar to chronic use of psychoactive drugs (Volkow et al., 2008). This reverse interpretation argues that the reduced pleasure in obese people is a consequence of overeating and obesity, rather its cause. Ironically, overeating results in a dull dopamine response, which makes food less satisfying and motivates even more eating to compensate. They are chasing the high or earlier pleasurable experience. Highly palatable foods have the capacity to rewire our brains (neuroadaptation), driving us to seek more of those products. As a result, people cannot control their responses to highly palatable foods because their brains have been changed by the foods they eat (Benton, 2010).

Similarly, use of addictive drugs eventually causes dopamine receptors to reduce in numbers (the tolerance and withdrawal mechanisms). Recent evidence supports this alternative view that the dopamine suppression might disappear once the excessive body weight or excessive reward consumption was stopped. Obese women weighing over 200 pounds who as a result of gastric bypass surgery lost about 25 pounds after 6 weeks produced a rise in their dopamine receptor levels, roughly proportional to the amount of weight loss (Steel et al., 2009). This evidence of a rise in dopamine level after weight loss is more consistent with the view that the obesity caused the lower level of dopamine receptors, rather than an innate dopamine deficit causing overeating.

---

[3]Similarly, individuals prone to abuse drugs have been found to have lower levels of dopamine concentration in neural pathways than those less prone to abuse drugs. As a result, they are more receptive to the reinforcing effects of drugs and other rewarding stimuli.

The direction of causality remains to be resolved. Is decreased sensitivity of the dopamine-reward a result of repeated overstimulation of the system, or is it a preexisting risk factor for obesity or drug abuse? It is possible that heightened dopamine release in reward centers is a risk factor for excessive food intake among normal weight individuals and that those who become overweight show a resulting down-regulation of dopamine receptors that produces a heightened need for food reward to reach an acceptable level of hedonic satisfaction.

Dopamine also plays an important role in inhibitory control. The mechanism by which lower D_2 receptors could increase overeating is the regulation of desire to eat. Lower dopamine availability is associated with lower activity in the prefrontal cortex, which contributes to inhibitory control. Evidence shows that individuals with the gene variant that is linked with lower D_2 receptor expression had lower inhibitory control than individuals with the gene variant associated with higher D_2 receptor expression (Volkow et al., 2008). These individuals are less likely to succeed in regulating their emotional reactions associated with strong desires (for drugs or food).

Summary

Dopamine plays an important role in motivation, reward, learning, and inhibition control that regulate eating behavior. Brain imaging studies show that obese individuals have significantly lower D_2 receptor levels, which make them less sensitive to reward stimuli, which in turn would make them more vulnerable to food intake as a means to temporarily compensate for this deficit. The decreased D_2 receptor levels are also associated with decreased inhibitory control that may influence the inability to control food intake in the obese individuals in the presence of highly palatable food.

It is possible that obese individuals anticipate greater reward from food intake and report greater reward from food intake. Preferences for high-fat and high-sugar foods predict elevated weight gain and increased risk of obesity. Intake of high-fat and high-sugar foods results in a low level of D_2 receptors. Thus, overeating may lead to receptor down-regulation, which may increase the likelihood of further overeating and continued weight gain (Lowe, van Steenburgh, Ochner, & Coletta, 2009).

It is also possible that the reduced dopamine receptors in obese individuals can be viewed as reducing all other life pleasures, so that food remains the only pleasure available for consumption (Berridge, 2007). Thus reduced dopamine receptors could be a consequence, not the cause, of sustained obesity. The process seems like a trap; the more you overeat unhealthy, high-sugar foods, the more you see a dampening of enjoyment, and the more you overcompensate by overeating. Such changes might help explain the notoriously high rate of diet failure.

THE OPPONENT-PROCESS MODEL

The two views discussed above are consistent with the *opponent-process model* developed by Solomon (1977). The model provides a model of transition to addiction. This model conceptualizes addiction as a disorder that progresses from impulsivity to compulsivity. The sources of motivation for the impulsive act include pleasure or relief during the act. Compulsive behavior (obsessive thoughts) is motivated to release negative emotions (anxiety and stress). The process involves the neurobiological change in brain reward homeostasis that may lead drug use to drug addiction and relapse.

The opponent-process model assumes that the central nervous system of mammals spontaneously opposes diverse types of affective or hedonic states. Any environmental factor that challenges homeostasis is hypothesized to be met with counter actions. Initially a stimulus, whether agreeable or aversive, leads to a primary affective reaction. This primary reaction is called *a-process*. The a-process will automatically activate a *b-process*, which opposes the initial reaction by producing an opposite reaction. This self-regulating process represents homeostasis.

Related to drug abuse, Solomon argued that the a-processes could reflect the intense rush of pleasure from drugs. These pleasurable effects disappear with repeated use and are replaced with aversive withdrawal symptoms, reflecting the b-processes and leading to craving. Once addiction has set in, the appetitive effects of drugs are of little importance as the individual becomes completely tolerant to them. Thus, the motive to use becomes to alleviate withdrawal symptoms. Koob and Le Moal (2005) suggest that the excessive utilization of a drug creates an overactivation of the brain reward system. In other words, the b-process may get progressively larger during intermittent drug taking. Therefore, initially addicts use drug for the positive hedonic effects, but later on addiction is motivated primarily by avoidance of negative hedonic state. With repeated drug use, the underlying opponent b-process increases in magnitude and duration, leading to an experience dominated by the unpleasant symptoms associated with withdrawal (Solomon & Corbit, 1973.)

THE INCENTIVE-SALIENCE THEORY

The *incentive-salience theory* (Berridge, 2009) provides another perspective by suggesting that changes in brain reward system are important for the transition from casual to compulsive drug use and food consumption.

Initially, many potentially addictive drugs produce feelings of euphoria and encouraging further use. However, repeated drug use (becoming addicted) appears to decrease the role of pleasure. Once addicted, the desire to use drugs (wanting) disproportionately exceeds the pleasure effect of drugs (liking). This dissociation between wanting and liking progressively increases with the development of addiction. It is commonly known that drug addicts report that they continue to crave their drug long after they have stopped enjoying it. This insight also provides another perspective on how a distorted reward system may contribute to compulsive overeating and obesity. For example, the sight or smell of food could trigger a compulsive urge to eat, even though the person would not derive higher pleasure from it.

According to the incentive salience theory, it is hypothesized that the process of reward consists of two components, that is, "liking" and "wanting." Normally liking and wanting go hand-in-hand: we want what we like and like what we want. However, the work by the psychologist Kent Berridge et al. (2009) suggests that liking and wanting might differ. In other words, the brain appears to generate "wanting" and "liking" via separable mechanisms. "Liking" refers to the pleasure that comes from actually tasting food. However, liking does not determine the incentive value of food. The incentive value of food is reflected by wanting it. "Wanting" refers to appetite or craving, or the anticipation of something delicious, which helps determine its motivational incentive value. "Wanting" is distinguishable from more cognitive forms of desire meant by the ordinary word, wanting. "Wanting" does not require elaborate cognitive expectations and is focused more directly on reward-related stimuli. Liking can be inferred from ratings of the palatability of food. Wanting can be inferred through behavioral measures of how hard a person will work to obtain food.

"Liking" and "wanting" are thought to be controlled by different brain mechanisms. With respect to food, opioids give food its pleasure, and dopamine motivates our behavior toward food. Thus, dopamine is less about pleasure and reward than about drive and motivation (Berridge, 2007). For example, elevated dopamine levels in the brain of mutant mice, whose gene mutation causes extra dopamine production, increased wanting for sweet rewards (Wang et al., 2001). Similarly, studies in humans have shown elevation of wanting without liking (Berridge, 2007). It is important to note that the elevation of dopamine levels triggers wanting for reward that leads to pursuit, rather than food overconsumption. However, once the consumption meal is begun, other (e.g., opioid) brain mechanisms could extend the amount of meal consumed.

In addiction theory, this pathological or hypersensitive motivation (wanting) is referred to as *sensitization*, which is an incentive caused by repeated drug use. The sensitization effect provides a mechanism to explain why addicts continue to want drugs and relapse even after long periods of abstinence. Evidence shows that addiction occupies an inordinate amount of an individual's time and thoughts and persists despite adverse consequences. For example, an addict with no drug may spend the day engaging in a series of behaviors, such as lying and stealing, to obtain the drug.

Learning plays a major role in the incentive model as it interacts with the wanting and liking dimension and thus directs motivation to specific and appropriate targets. There are two types of learning: *reward expectancy* and *associative learning*. When we learn that a stimulus provides gratification, the knowledge drives our wanting and our anticipation of feeling better. For example, consider a person who habitually consumes certain foods to relieve unpleasant emotions. The relief of stress produced by the food is encoded in the memory. A strong memory trace is thus formed between stress relief and food consumption. Later, when encountering a stressful situation, the memory is activated, culminating in the experience of craving and wanting. Moreover, stress could contribute to binge eating when stress and food cues combine together. In short, learned associations promote habitual behaviors with little conscious recognition (Berridge, Ho, Richard, & DiFeliceantonio, 2010).

The key to which stimulus becomes "wanted" may lie in Pavlovian learning mechanisms. For example, repeated presentation of a palatable food is likely to induce strong Pavlovian conditioning, creating conditioned stimuli that strongly activate dopamine systems more than in an individual that has not undergone the same conditioning experience. Wanting system is more sensitive to the widespread availability of highly palatable food, which creates hedonic hunger ("perceived deprivation"). Cue-triggered "wanting" does not need to be conscious and are triggered by relatively basic stimuli and perceptions. The difference between "wanting" and more cognitive desires can sometimes lead to what could be called irrational "wanting" for outcomes that are not cognitively wanted and that are neither liked nor even expected to be liked. Obese individuals report stronger craving of high-fat, high-sugar foods than lean individuals. They also work harder for food and are more likely to eat in the absence of hunger.

The insight from the incentive theory provides a better understanding of how distorted "wanting" may produce compulsive overeating and a possible mechanism for food addiction[4] (Finlayson, King, & Blundell, 2007).

---

[4]It is important to note that food liking and wanting can dissociate somewhat even in normal situations. Liking and wanting vary in graded fashion along a continuum, rather than of kind. The discrepancy between wanting and liking can lead to bad decisions. For example, buying exercise equipment, joining a health club, and compulsive shopping, where there is a possible disconnection between the wanting of these goods and the liking from consuming them.

If eating disorders involve a pathology in some aspect of brain reward function, such as an excessive "wanting" system, it would be possible that such an individual would "want" to eat food at the same time that they cognitively do not want to eat, and when "liking" would not be enhanced. In other words, the sight, smell, or vivid imagination of food could trigger a compulsive urge to eat, even though the person would not expect to find the experience very pleasurable. For example, Stice et al. (2010) report that obese people appear not to get as much pleasure as they expect from tasty treats. These findings somewhat contradict the popular notion that overweight people love to eat and get more pleasure than others out of rich treats. In other words, obese individuals expect more reward but seem to experience less.

In sum, the evidence supports the idea that obese individuals overeat to compensate for the mismatch they experience between their strong cravings (wanting) and the reduced enjoyment (liking) they get. The best way to avoid this vicious circle is to develop healthy eating habits, before pleasure responses get blunted by overeating.

TRAIT IMPULSIVITY

The trait of impulsiveness may be another important individual variable in identifying those most vulnerable to overeating and weight gain. Individual differences in one's susceptibility to impulses and ability to exercise inhibitory control is recognized as a major risk factor in vulnerability to drug abuse and obesity. People with an impulsive personality are simply more prone to be impulsive and they overeat more easily.

The measurement of time preference captures aspects of personality traits. Factors such as deliberation, difficulty to think about consequences, and the capacity to inhibit impulses likely determine discount factors or time preferences more generally. As discussed in Chapter 6, delay discounting is the measure of how much an individual is driven by immediate gratification versus the willingness to wait for delayed but greater rewards. Thus, the higher discounting may be tapping into a trait that is a factor leading to development of obesity. There is some evidence that shows higher delay discounting in obese individuals (Davis et al., 2007). Obese individuals show a preference for smaller, immediate rewards, rather than larger delayed rewards, indicating poor and impulsive decision making. For example, as compared with healthy-weight women, obese women selected more immediate choices than delayed choices of greater value on a delay discounting of money task, suggesting greater impulsivity (Davis et al., 2004). Another study (Weller, Cook, Avsar, & Cox, 2008) found that obese women display significantly weaker impulse control than normal-weight women, but between obese and normal-weight men, the impulsivity levels are nearly the same.[5] Impulsivity makes it more difficult for some individuals to resist the temptation to eat too much and can thereby contribute to overweight (Guerrieri et al., 2007). In general, more impulsive individuals may have more difficulty stopping themselves from eating palatable foods or eating in response to emotion, which could then contribute to weight gain or to making weight loss more difficult.

Impulsivity is also associated with higher weight in children. Obese children are more likely to behave impulsively than children of normal weight (Guerrieri et al., 2007). They are less able to delay gratification and more often choose a direct reward over a larger delayed reward. Overweight versus lean children consume more calories after exposure to food cues, such as smelling and tasting a palatable food, suggesting that the former are more likely to give in to cravings resulting from food cues.

Impulsivity, however, is not a homogenous construct but rather consists of a number of dimensions. The term impulsivity is typically defined as the tendency to respond immediately without thinking about consequences, the inability to delay gratification or tolerate boredom, and the tendency to seek out novel or exciting stimuli. The various facets of impulsivity are related to two specific factors: *reward sensitivity* (a tendency to exaggerate the impact of reward) and *self-control ability*. Reward sensitivity may contribute to greater sensitivity and attention toward food-related cues and subsequent craving, purchasing, and preparing of binge food. Self-control, on the other hand, may be reflected in loss of control over eating during binge episodes or the inability to resist binge craving.

Furthermore, the two factors have separate biological bases. Each of these responses is supported by a specific brain network. Reward sensitivity is supported by the dopamine system, and the prefrontal cortex is involved in self-control behavior. Studies (Davis et al., 2007) have suggested deficits in executive function/inhibitory control in obese individuals. The slow activation in executive system regions may lead to decisions being driven more by other systems (i.e., reward), resulting in relatively more choices for immediate compared with delayed rewards. This may lead to an obesogenic pattern of food choices focusing on immediate gratification rather than long-term health considerations.

---

[5]One explanation for the differences between men and women may be found in a personality trait known as eating-related disinhibition, which is the tendency to overeat in response to certain situations or cues, such as a big display of dessert. Men score lower in disinhibition than women.

In sum, impulsivity is a key component of decision-making deficits. Impulsive behavior may result from increased drive for pleasure or reward, decreased inhibitory ability, or both. An impulsivity component of personality may be a risk factor for the development of binge-eating and obesity. The tendency to overeat can lead to the development of unhealthy strategies to control weight, such as skipping meals, which may explain why obese individuals develop eating disorders.

OVEREATING AND POOR DECISION MAKING

We are constantly confronted with decisions about whether to consume food in light of its long-term benefits or hazards. Poor decision making is most prominently seen in drug addiction. Decision-making impairments are related to deficits in prefrontal cortex. Addicts tend to choose actions that bring immediate reward, even when this leads to a deleterious outcome at some later date. Thus, in pathological overeating (such as binge eating), functions of the prefrontal cortex may play an important role in the maintenance of binge attacks.

How do people make eating decisions? As discussed in the previous chapter, the dual-system model describes a person's decision as the product of two separate, but interacting systems[6]: (1) an impulsive system for signaling the pain or pleasure of the immediate prospects of an option; and (2) a reflective system for signaling the pain or pleasure of the future prospects of an option (Bechara, 2005). The impulsive system gets things done quickly (i.e., emotional reactions arising from relatively automatic processes) but is prone to error. It involves slowly learned associations over an accumulated set of experience and requires minimal cognitive resources. In contrast, the reflective system is driven by thoughts and reflection. The reflective system can learn rules using language and logic. It is relatively more controlled and involved in thinking, reasoning, and consciousness. Like a watchful parent, the reflective system's goal is to rein in our impulses and override our snap judgments. The final decision is determined by the relative strengths of these two systems. For example, when the immediate prospect is unpleasant but the future is

---

[6]Individuals with pathology in decision making are part of the same population considered clinically normal. For example, everyone experiences anxiety, but patients with trait anxiety suffer from a level of anxiety that incapacitates them. The anxiety continuum stretches between two poles, each of which is pathological. One pole is characteristic of the antisocial personality who is deprived of anxiety even in the most dangerous situations. The other pole is characteristic of highly emotional individuals whose chronic anxiety debilitates them.

more pleasant, then the positive signal of future prospects forms the basis for enduring the unpleasantness of the immediate prospect. When the immediate prospects dominate, the decision shifts toward short-term horizons.[7]

There are at least two underlying types of dysfunction where this overall signal turns in favor of immediate outcomes: (1) hyperactivity in the impulsive system, which exaggerates the rewarding impact of available incentives, such as food; and (2) hypoactivity in the prefrontal cortex or reflective system, which forecasts the long-term consequences of a given action. Obese individuals may be afflicted with either one or both of those dysfunctions (Volkow et al., 2008).

In the case of food addiction, the individual becomes unable to choose according to long-term outcomes, which require that the pain/pleasure signals triggered by the reflective system dominate those from the impulsive system. Two broad types of conditions could alter this relationship and lead to loss of willpower: (1) a dysfunctional reflective system that has lost its ability to process the future prospects; and (2) a hyperactive impulsive system that exaggerates the immediate prospects. This increased strength of the impulsive system can alter the balance of power in favor of impulsive system. This in turn will bias or even "hijack" the cognitive mechanisms needed for the normal operation of the reflective system. This is why, from the perspective of someone who is dieting and has lost the willpower to resist a tempting food, the decision to eat that food becomes very reasonable and logical at the time of consumption.

As noted before, the most clearly established commonality of the mechanisms of food and drug intake is that they both exert their reinforcing effects partly by increasing dopamine in the brain reward system. The enhanced activation of the dopamine system increases preference for the intake of foods high in fat and sugar, even in animals fed beyond apparent satiety (Kelley, 2004). The enhanced sensitivity in the reward system sensitizes the impulsive system by increasing the desire, urge, or motivation to seek the rewarding food item. The activation of the impulsive system may impact the prefrontal cortex functions, so that it can undermine the cognitive capacity for exerting inhibitory control to resist calorie-rich food items (Naqvi & Bechara, 2009).

---

[7]The dual-system decision model can be interpreted naturally as the behavioral manifestation of a conflict between two selves: one inclined to consume more today, the other inclined to save for the future. The key idea of dual-self model is the conflict between the two selves. The short-run preference is assumed to be located in the limbic system and the long-run preferences in the lateral prefrontal cortex.

The prefrontal cortex[8] controls skills such as regulation of affective impulses and inhibition of behavioral actions. The right prefrontal cortex appears to play a critical role in behavioral restraint and self-control by keeping reward-generating mechanisms in check. Damage to the right frontal cortex can lead to a general disregard for the long-term adverse consequences of behavioral choice, such as excessive food intake (Alonso-Alonso & Pascual-Leone, 2007). For instance, successful dieters who have significantly higher levels of dietary restraint in comparison with non-dieters show increased neural activity in the right prefrontal cortex in response to food consumption (Del Parigi et al., 2007; Kuijer, de Ridder, Ouwehand, Houx, & van den Bos, 2008).

Much of the early research on decision making came from studying the social impairments of patients with ventromedial prefrontal cortical (VMPFC) lesions, and the observation that their behavioral deficits are typically caused by an inability to advantageously assess future consequences.[9] Patients with damage to ventral and medial parts of the prefrontal cortex (PFC) show impairments in motivated behavior (Bechara, 2005). The classic case is that of Phineas Gage (Damasio, 1994) who experienced a severe, penetrating injury to the ventromedial frontal cortex. In spite of relatively preserved cognitive function, Gage appeared to lose his ability to make advantageous decisions where the decision process involved weighing costs and benefits. Gage's social function was profoundly affected and he was no longer motivated by social norms, suggesting disrupted reward function. Damasio (1996), following careful observation of similar patients, formulated the concept of *somatic marker hypothesis*. The theory suggests that signaling the prospective consequences of options for choice can assist in selection of advantageous decision making. However, patients with ventromedial prefrontal lesions do not make advantageous decisions because they lack the ability to incorporate predictions regarding the emotional consequences of an action into the decision proves.

Studies (Bechara, 2005) have shown that some addicts closely resemble VMPFC lesion patients; that is, they show insensitivity to future consequences, both positive and negative. These impairments have also been found in bulimia nervosa patients, and in obese women (Davis, Strachan, & Berkson, 2004). Research shows that abnormalities in the reflective system involved in inhibitory control may also contribute to

---

[8]Research suggests that affect in the human brain is controlled primarily by the PFC (Lowe et al., 2009). Within the PFC, there exist at least three separable neural systems: the orbitofrontal, ventromedial, and dorsolateral cortices, all of which are involved in affect regulation, complex goal-directed behavior, and feeding.
[9]The ventromedial PFC is a subdivision of the PFC.

obesity (Davis et al., 2007).[10] The abnormality in the reflective system in obese individuals can lead to a general disregard for the long-term adverse consequences of behavioral choice (e.g., gaining weight, diabetes). They are less likely to succeed in inhibiting the temptations to eat high-calorie food. Women suffering from eating disorders are often well aware of the adverse consequences of ongoing binge attacks and often feel ashamed about them. Especially in periods preceding a binge attack, however, they lack the ability to make advantageous decisions. Even though they may evaluate risks cognitively, they react to them emotionally (Loewenstein, Weber, Hsee, & Welch, 2001). Emotional reactions are largely dependent on proximity in time and place. In other words, even though binge eaters may cognitively consider the risks of overeating, they still make inappropriate choices because they may be more influenced by the rewarding values of readily available foods.

However, it is not clear whether impulsive responding is a precursor to addiction disorders or whether it only occurs because of the brain alterations caused by excessive use. Research (Verdejo-Garcia et al., 2004) shows that the developmental VMPFC malfunction does not cause addiction; rather, it provides a risk factor that tends to render individuals "myopic" for future consequences and, therefore, more likely to be guided in the direction of immediately gratifying behaviors, such as drug taking.

Attentional Bias

Attentional bias is the allocation of the user's attention to substance-related stimuli[11] (Figure 9.1). It is defined as an exaggerated amount of attention given to highly rewarding foods. Accumulated evidence suggests that

FIGURE 9.1   Attentional Bias

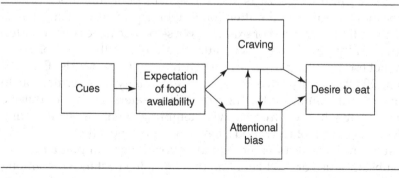

---

[10]Impairment in the reflective system, including memory, abstract reasoning, and attention, is also associated with an increased body weight in adults (Gunstad et al., 2007). This association may exist as early as in childhood: overweight children and children at risk for overweight have decreased mental ability compared with normal-weight children (Li et al., 2008).
[11]Dopamine derives desire through a survival-based capacity known as "attentional bias."

addictive behavior is characterized by biases in the attentional processing of drug-related stimuli. These drug cues acquire the ability to grab the user's attention. Field and Cox (2008) present a theoretical framework to explain how attentional bias develops and how it is related to important aspects of addictive behaviors.

The diagram shows that through classical conditioning,[12] food-related cues elicit the expectancy of food availability, and this expectancy causes both attentional bias for food-related cues and craving. As discussed before, repeated use of a substance of abuse produces a dopaminergic response that becomes sensitized. These cues are flagged as "salient," and they grab the users' attention. Consequently, the sensitized dopamine system produces both craving and attentional bias that motivates drug-seeking behavior.

Attentional bias and craving are mutually related such that increases in one lead to increases in the other, a process that is likely to result in overeating. That is, when food-related cues become the focus of attention, subjective craving increases. This, in turn, increases the attention-grabbing properties of food-related cues. Once the addict becomes aware of the craving, he or she "elaborates" on it, for example, by ruminating on the craving itself or maintaining attentional focus on the cues that triggered it. The elaboration, in turn, increases the strength of the subjective craving. As craving increases, reward-related stimuli will become more salient, and as the reward-related cues become the focus of attention, they will elicit further increases in subjective craving.

Impulsivity and impaired self-control appear to influence the strength of attentional biases and craving. Addicts with poor inhibitory control will have difficulty inhibiting their responses to substance-related stimuli. Thus, highly impulsive addicts and those with poor inhibitory control might be more sensitive to the attention-grabbing properties of substance-related stimuli than others. For example, obese people have been reported to automatically direct their visual attention more to the sight of foods than nonobese people, particularly when hungry (Nijs, Muris, Euser, & Franken, 2009). Obesity involves greater externality or overreaction to incentive stimuli. Similarly, the high-restrained eaters that are impulsive would overeat when confronted with tempting foods, or in tempting situations (e.g., smell of tasty foods, food exposure, and a typical preload).

In sum, individual differences in attentional bias can predict subsequent substance use or the likelihood of relapse to substance use among

---

[12]According to classical conditioning, a substance-related cue acquires motivational properties that produce craving. For example, pairing of the rewarding effects of alcohol with the sight and smell of vodka consistently increases cravings.

individuals who are attempting to abstain. Knowledge about attentional bias has important implications for diet relapse avoidance. For example, dieters might use cognitive avoidance strategies in an attempt to suppress their food craving and involuntary attentional processing of food-related stimuli.

Affect Regulation

The *affect regulation* model of binge eating suggests binge eaters use food to cope with stress and other negative feelings to regulate their emotions. Eating palatable foods relieves stress or anxiety by increasing pleasant feelings. Binge eating may be used as a means to escape from these negative feelings. These negative feelings temporarily increase the relative rewarding values of certain foods. Negative feelings also deplete one's limited self-control resources required in regulating one's emotions. However, the effect is short-lived and followed by shame or guilt and other negative feelings. An increased BMI could lead to more frequent periods of depressed mood and, therefore, more overeating.

Thus, individuals with abnormalities in food reward, those who believe that eating reduces negative affect and enhances positive affect, would be more likely to use food as a means to repair negative feelings. Evidence shows that women with binge eating disorder do have difficulties regulating emotions in daily life and adopt unhealthy emotion-regulation strategies. Several studies (Svaldi, Brand, & Tuschen-Caffier, 2010; Whiteside et al., 2007) show the potential role of affect-regulation deficits in the maintenance of the binge eating disorder. To reduce binge episodes, cognitive behavioral therapy (CBT) provides a useful and a more affect regulation skills to encounter triggers identified as predisposing to binge attacks.

CONCLUSION

Excessive overeating can disturb brain reward mechanisms in a manner similar to that caused by addictive drug abuse. Chronic overeating causes down-regulation of dopamine levels to compensate for its overstimulation. This increases the "wanting" of food, even if the enjoyment associated with its consumption diminishes. As food begins to take on greater incentive value, it also becomes less resistible and more able to control an individual's behavior.

Trait impulsivity is strongly associated with compulsive overeating and binge eating. Overweight and obese people seem more sensitive to reward and less adequate at the inhibition of temptation, especially when it comes to resisting palatable food. This suggests that those who are highly sensitive to the rewarding properties of food and who are "myopic" about the future negative consequences of a diet are more likely to make poor food choices. Thus, effective treatments need to address problem-solving and decision-making skills to improve impulse control.

The addiction framework provides a new paradigm for addressing the obesity issue. The most important implication is that the widespread availability and aggressive advertising of unhealthy foods may undermine public health interventions to decrease consumption of these foods. Constant confrontation with palatable food may inevitably trigger the desire to eat. This accessibility, in combination with our innate preferences for palatable foods, can be used to exploit vulnerable individuals and to increase the likelihood that people will abuse food, in much the same way that addicts misuse other addictive substances. Thus, public policy interventions designed to limit exposure to unhealthy foods for both adults and children may prove to be effective in reducing excess food consumption.

Since the development of addiction involves multiple brain systems (i.e., reward, motivation, learning, memory, and inhibitory control), the prevention and treatment of obesity should be comprehensive and use a multimodal approach. Similar to substance dependence, effective approaches for food addiction and obesity treatments include identification of triggers and other relapse prevention strategies. Strategies aimed at improving brain dopamine function might be beneficial in the treatment and prevention of obesity. These strategies include decreasing the rewarding properties of the food; enhancing the rewarding properties of alternative behaviors (i.e., social interactions, physical activity); disrupting the conditioned-learned associations (i.e., promoting new habits to substitute for old ones); and strengthening self-control, as discussed in Chapter 11.

There is now a range of available medications for each of the major classes of addictive drugs, which, in combination with psychotherapy or counseling, have been effective in reducing the likelihood of relapse. One mechanism for the success of these drugs seems to be their ability to diminish the strong urges and craving-associated addiction disorders. For example, Naltrexone is an anticraving medication that regulates the release of dopamine in reward pathways. This drug has been used successfully in the treatment of opiate addiction and alcoholism. In sum, successful obesity treatments require that we need to develop interventions that will (1) decrease activation of impulsive brain regions and (2) increase activity in executive brain regions. This can be accomplished by exercising cognitive control or medication to compensate for decision failures.

Clinical experience suggests that patients with binge eating disorder often report an overemphasis on food as the only source of enjoyment in their lives. On the other hand, negative emotions are also major triggers for both binge eating and substance use, since food and drugs can dull or distract from emotional distress. Recognition of these factors points to the importance of helping binge eating disorder patients find alternative sources of reward and pleasure in their lives besides food and eating.

Drug addiction and compulsive overeating also require the interruption of learned habits. Both behaviors are conditioned responses to certain triggers and are generally followed by highly rewarding consequences. Use of cue management strategies, such as limiting the availability of "binge foods," may be helpful. As in drug addiction, the consumption of binge foods, typically high-calorie, high-fat foods, has a priming[13] effect that can trigger compulsive overeating (Volkow & Wise, 2005). Thus, avoiding trigger foods is the recommended course of action. The effective treatment approach involves efforts to break the bond between the conditioned stimuli (food cues) and the unconditioned stimuli (eating). Such a treatment consists of repeated presentations of the rewarding food cues while eating (the response) is prevented. Moreover, overcoming an addiction requires an individual to learn to tolerate negative emotional states, including cravings and urges, without acting on them (Dingemans, Martijn, Jansen, & van Furth, 2009). That is why the development of emotion regulation and distress tolerance skills could be central to the treatment of both BED and drug addiction.

As discussed before, the two hypothesized brain systems, impulsive system ("go") and self-controlled system ("stop"), are often in conflict. They are moderated by a variety of punishments and rewards imposed by the environments as well as personality traits. For example, sedentary behaviors are widely rewarded in the modern society, whereas they would have been punished in a hunter-gatherer society. Similarly, in the past highly palatable foods were not readily available, so there was a survival advantage to overeating when such foods were available. However, the abundant availability of cheap palatable foods in most developed societies continually challenges our cognitive capacity to control the evolutionarily driven impulse to eat.[14] This is especially problematic for those vulnerable individuals who exhibit impulsivity and sensitivity to reward.

---

[13]The fact that binge eating is often triggered by the ingestion of small amounts of a palatable food parallels the "priming" effect of drugs in addicts, whereby the initial ingestion of the drug tends to elicit a strong "craving" or compulsion for further use.

[14]As noted previously, the obesity issue partly stems from the fact that we have kept the eating habits of our ancestors with a modern lifestyle.

Given the high availability of palatable food, the need to control one's impulse in stimulus-intense settings becomes increasingly important. More than ever before in our history, the maintenance of a healthy body weight seems dependent on the strength of the prefrontal cortex necessary for making good decisions overriding the strength of the drive to consume calories. The ability to resist temptations may require skills such as behavior inhibition, attention shift, and delay of gratification. Hence, the ability to make advantageous decisions may increase the likelihood of overeating.

10

Why Dieters Relapse

INTRODUCTION

Relapse, temporary loss of control and return to old behavior, is common in dieting. Despite documented short-term success, dieting has a very low success rates; most dieters regain their weight back within 3–5 years[1] (Institute of Medicine [IOM], (2003). The question is why do people fail to stick to a healthy diet in order to lose weight? This chapter addresses the question of what factors make weight loss maintenance so difficult. It describes the mechanisms underlying diet relapse. The chapter presents some insights from behavioral economics to explain why people fail to maintain healthy behaviors. Knowing why people fail to maintain a desired preference for healthy behavior over time is an essential ingredient in the development of effective weight-loss management.

FACTORS INFLUENCING DIET RELAPSE

Dieting behavior can be viewed as making constant trade-offs between immediate and delayed benefits under uncertain conditions. This difference in the timing of costs and benefits constitutes one of the major obstacles to dieting (Herman & Polivy, 2002). Diets have consequences, which are realized only after long periods of time, and they typically involve incurring a current cost in exchange for the chance of some future benefit. In order to attain the long-term goal of weight loss, dieters must be able to consistently resist the immediate temptation of food. This will require the dieter to resist preference change and satisfy current preference. The success in dieting requires the individual to impose current preferences on the future.[2]

---

[1]The research firm Marketdata Enterprises shows that the dieting industry earned $55 billion in 2006 and is expected to rise to $68.7 billion in 2010. Diet programs such as Weight Watchers and Jenny Craig made $1.2 billion and $462 million, respectively, in 2006.
[2]It is important to note that physiological changes (e.g., decreases in metabolic rate) that occur during weight loss can promote weight regain.

At any point in time, one's preferences depend not only on stable factors but also on transient factors that cause preferences to change rapidly from moment to moment. There are several mechanisms that are capable of generating temporary preference reversals. The following sections enumerate a number of choice situations that tend to interfere with dieters' resolve to diet and induce them to become impulsive.[3] Under these conditions, the dieter gives too little weight to the future consequences relative to the immediate benefits. These situations are most commonly seen as the struggle between impulses and restraints, which require self-control to protect the person's overarching goal. If these choice situations occur repeatedly, preference reversals could have a large cumulative impact.

Hunger

Hunger plays a critical role in intertemporal choice (Loewenstein, 1996). Hunger triggers a negative emotional response that leads people to become impatient.[4] To be hungry is to be uncomfortable, and most of us experience hunger in the same way we experience pain—as a signal to do something. Suddenly all other concerns fall away. People become combative or aggressive[5] when they are hungry (Crockett, Clark, Robbins, Tabibnia, & Lieberman, 2008). As people get hungrier, less attention is given to healthy diets. Hunger promotes eating not by increasing the desirability of the food but by reducing the dieter's will or ability to resist. Thus, the intentions to follow a healthy diet can be thwarted by hunger (Tomiyama, Mann, & Comer, 2009).

It is said that hunger is the best spice. We will enjoy our lunch more for being deprived of breakfast. For example, hunger makes sweetness taste more pleasant, and satiety reduces the same sensation of pleasantness. Endogenous opioid activation is a chief candidate to make food taste better during hunger. Thus, when one is hungry, food becomes extra rewarding, which leads to overeating. This also explains why treating obesity by restricting diet is often unsuccessful (Stice, Yokum, Blum, & Bohon, 2010). Interventions that

---

[3]It is not clear whether chronic dieters are all prone to disinhibited eating in certain situations or only some of them are prone to disinhibited eating. This question will not be addressed here.

[4]Hunger is a learned behavior and could be viewed as an addiction (Hebb, 1949). Similar to addiction, food cues become conditioned and develop the ability to induce craving, approach, and consumption. Conditioned cues paired with food intakes promote dopamine release.

[5]The essential amino acid necessary for the body to create serotonin (tryptophan) can only be obtained through eating. Our serotonin levels naturally decline when we don't eat. Eating tryptophan-rich foods, such as poultry (chicken soup) and chocolate, can boost serotonin levels (perhaps this is why these are called "feel good" foods).

reduce hunger might be more effective if they aim to reduce feelings of hunger. Findings from the National Weight Control Registry[6] suggest that a key component of successful weight loss maintenance is eating breakfast every day (Wing & Phelan, 2005). By eating regularly, people can avoid situations that encourage overeating. Mancino and Kinsey (2004) suggest that decreasing the interval between meals would reduce caloric intake by 45 calories a day. Over a year, this would result in a about a five pound reduction in total body weight, all else being equal. One way to mitigate the hunger problem would be to plan ahead and make food choices before increasing vulnerability to hunger.

Hedonic Hunger

Dieters may eat less than they would like to eat, rather than eating less than they need to eat to maintain energy balance. *Restrained eaters,*[7] relative to unrestrained eaters, are prone to feelings of hedonic deprivation because they sometimes avoid eating the amount of food, or the types of food, they would like to eat. Lowe and Butryn (2007) have suggested that being chronically tempted by palatable foods in the environment while trying to resist those temptations could create a state of *hedonic hunger* (or *perceived deprivation*). They suggest that the presence of food may stimulate psychological hunger just as the absence of food causes physiological hunger, especially when one eats less than is desired. Individuals who experience perceived deprivation more often may be at heightened risk for future weight gain. In the battle between appetitive drives to consume more palatable food than one needs and the conscious resistance to this drive, appetite often wins (Lowe, 2003). It is thus not surprising that in a society saturated with food cues, dieters have difficulty losing weight. Even when people are successful at losing weight, the long-term outcome for the vast majority is that they regain the weight they lost.

Stress

Hunger, of course, is not the only reason people eat. Stress, boredom and pleasure all come into play. We live in a world that entices us to relax and eat—a lot. There is a strong association between stress, mood,

---

[6]The National Weight Control Registry is a database of more than 4,000 individuals who have lost at least 10% of their body weight and kept it off at least one year. http://www.nwcr.ws/default.htm

[7]Restrained eaters are chronic dieters who want to reduce or at least maintain their present weight.

and increased eating. Loneliness, boredom, anxiety, depression, hectic schedules,[8] family crises, and personal conflicts lead to the urge to raid the refrigerator. People typically respond to stress by increasing their intake of readily available "comfort foods" loaded with sugar and fat (i.e., chocolate). Dallman, Pecoraro, and la Fleur (2005) show that the tendency to overeat in the face of chronic stress is biologically driven. Stress hormones stimulate appetite and the salience of rewards. They tell the brain, go get the goodies. It can be comfort food or other rewards, such as like drugs or sex. In a laboratory study (Dallman et al., 2005), when scientists added stress hormones to rats' brains, the animals remained stressed. But when they fed them sugar, the animals calmed down. When life is not going so smoothly and people reach for goodies full of fat and sugar, they are doing more than surrendering to cravings. Comfort foods like chocolate cake and ice cream literally blunt the body's response to chronic stress. A key critical predictor of relapse is the individual's ability to utilize effective coping strategies with stressful situations. Previous studies (Stroebe, 2008) document that overeating or binge eating focuses attention away from the stressful event, or enhances mood and thus counters the negative effects of stress on mood. Thus, distressed dieters overate because concerns for diet appear unimportant compared with the event that caused the emotional upheaval. Baumeister, Heatherton, and Tice (1994) argue that emotional arousal has the effect of narrowing attention to the most perceptually salient stimuli (e.g., food) and drawing attention away from broader and more abstract concerns (such as dieting). For example, a person may be dieting successfully in the hope of looking good in a swimsuit next summer—but intense emotional distress makes next summer seem impossibly far away and hence irrelevant, whereas consuming that entire cheesecake holds the (possibly illusory) promise of feeling better in the next few minutes. The distressed dieter experiences a disruption in her motivation to abstain and no longer cares so much about distant and doubtful goals. Short-term gratification replaces long-term objectives at the top of the motive hierarchy, and the result, especially in the presence of attractive food, is indulgence.[9] Dieters usually come to regret this decision, once the food is eaten, guilt is added to whatever distress obtained initially (Herman & Polivy, 2002).

---

[8]Research suggests that lack of sleep may lead to an increase in production of the hormone that stimulates appetite.

[9]Another explanation is the "escape from self-awareness" theory. Failure experiences and other threats to their ego or self-esteem are likely to motivate dieters to escape from self-awareness, which, in turn, undermines their motivation to monitor food intake.

Willpower

In general, willpower refers to effortful control that is exerted with the purpose of controlling our own behavior. Willpower is a resource that can be used to decrease or eliminate discrepancies between emotionally motivated and deliberatively desired behaviors. When people exert willpower or self-control, they inhibit their normal, typical, or automatic behavior. So, willpower depletion provides an alternative explanation for apparent intertemporal preference reversals. Dieters normally use willpower to restrain what they eat; stress weakens their restraints and they overeat. Successful dieters score highly on mental effort used to control weight (Graham & Wing, 2009). They deliberately eat small portions, avoid certain foods, count calories, and maintain a consistent diet across the week and year (including holidays).

Stress affects one's ability to maintain one's resolution to eat well. Coping with stress involves using mental processes and willpower to control behavior (Marlatt & Witkiewitz, 2005). Cognitive load is another factor that produces impulsive behavior. Imposing working memory load increases individuals' preferences for smaller, sooner rewards over larger, later ones. Boon, Stroebe, Schut, and Ijntema (2002) found that during distraction, dieters ate more of a "forbidden" food than when not distracted. Cognitive load interferes with dieters' monitoring of their food intake. Thus, the busier people are, the more likely they may be to behave impulsively.

Evidence shows that people who diet for personal reasons tend to be more successful at losing weight than people who diet for external reasons (Muraven, 2008). When a person resists eating sweets because dieting is valuable to him or her, it may require less self-control strength than when a person avoids eating a cookie because he or she was ordered to do so. Autonomous self-control may involve less feelings of internal conflict and may be more energizing than compelled self-control. Thus, making choices that feels autonomous leads to less depletion and better self-control performance than making choices when one feels forced.

Projection Bias

Projection bias is defined as falsely projecting current transient preferences on to the future. For instance, people in hot states (e.g., craving) tend to overestimate how long those states will last, a phenomenon that Loewenstein and O'Donoghue (2003) refer to as a "hot-to-cold empathy gap," or "projection bias." When in a cold state (e.g., satiated), we do not appreciate how much our desires and our behavior will be altered when we are hungry or craving ("under the influence"). For example, when a dieter is very hungry and appetizing aromas are emanating from the kitchen, we can say he or she is in a hot state. When he or she is thinking in abstract on Friday about the dinner on Saturday, he or she is in a cold state.

People tend to underappreciate the effects of changes in their states and hence falsely project their current preferences over consumption onto their future preferences. People in a cold state mispredict how they will behave in a hot state. When in a cold state (i.e., not hungry), it is difficult to imagine what it would feel like to be in a hot state or to imagine how one might behave in such a state. Likewise, when in a hot state (i.e., craving), people have difficulty imaging themselves in a cold state and thus miscalculate the speed with which such a state will dissipate. This concept supports the age-old folk wisdom that shopping on an empty stomach leads people to buy too much. People who are hungry act as if their future taste for food will reflect such hunger. For example, Read and Van Leeuwen (1998) reported that people who chose a snack they would not get for a week were more likely to choose an unhealthy snack if they were hungry when choosing than if they were not. This suggests that people were projecting their current tastes onto their future tastes. If people cannot imagine how overpowering the temptation will be, they cannot be expected to take protective action to avoid the tempting situations. To avoid this bias, one would be better off not to have impulse foods in the house, or eat before you shop, use a list, and stick to the perimeter of the store. That is where the fresh foods hang out.

Habit Formation

People are creatures of habit. Most people have routines that determine when they eat and how much they eat. Thus, if one's lifestyle supports a stable weight, one's weight is unlikely to change unless a person dramatically changes his or her lifestyle. Consumption over time leads to the accumulation of consumption capital stocks, similar to durable capital stock (Becker, 1992). Habits are a form of slowly accrued automaticity that involves the direct association between a context and a response. Habits are performed without any explicit goal. This explains the difficulty of making a smoking cessation choice after many years of smoking (and accumulating a large consumption stock).

Habit is generally reversible, in the sense that it depreciates (decays) unless maintained. Consistent nonreward will cause appetite to extinguish. In other words, if you do not satisfy the desire, it gets weaker to some extent.[10] Hence, it is plausible, if you crave donuts every day but

---

[10]The Roman physician Galen already knew this, pointing out that anger was tamed like a horse, but that the strong desire, like a wild boar or goat, had to be controlled by starvation.

never get them, the craving may dwindle and disappear. So refraining from indulgence may be the most reliable pathway to the abatement of desire. The desire does not vanish entirely, but may diminish. In the same way, the experiences of those so called successful losers show that weight maintenance gets easier with time. With time, the odds of regaining weight go down (Squires, 2005). People who maintain their new weight for 2 years have a greater likelihood of keeping it off for two more years (Wing & Phelan, 2005). Those who maintain it for 5 years have even greater odds of maintaining their weight loss. Once you have the habit, you would not think of not doing it. The behavior becomes automatic with practice (like driving a car).

Cue-Elicited Behavior

Psychologists call cue-elicited behavior "conditioned responses." Conditioned responses are built up through repetitive associations between cues and a particular consumption activity. Cues like the smell of cookies baking or the sight of a bowl of ice cream will induce craving in a dieter to order something sweet, reversing an earlier resolution to avoid the extra calories. The habit formation effects are turned on and off by the presence or absence of environmental cues (i.e., sensory inputs) (Laibson, 2001). Exposure to food cues induces conditioned physiological reactivity, which can prepare the person for the intake of food. This explains why those preferences often vary from moment to moment. Cues initiate physiological changes that prime[11] and creates craving for immediate consumption. Consequently, delaying consumption becomes costly.

The natural tendency is to underestimate the impact of food cues. It is recommended that dieters distance themselves from food cues that threaten their resolve: keep snack foods out of view, or stop buying foods where "you can't eat just one"; or remove themselves from food cues (going for long walks). Distancing oneself from cues that threaten one's resolve is a general tactic for enhancing one's willpower (Hoch & Lowenstein, 1991). A large literature shows that the availability of only limited types of foods (and thus limited food cues) causes reduced eating during a meal (Raynor & Epstein, 2001). Thus, simply removing the cues prevents us from overeating.[12]

---

[11]Priming refers to processes that increase the cognitive salience of stimuli.
[12]Since dieters tend to have limited variety in their diet, they may become bored on the restricted diets and may be highly responsive to palatable foods cues.

The Impact of Dietary Violations on Eating

In general, biological boundaries determine when a person feels hungry or satiated and thereby when a person starts and stops eating. People not on a diet are assumed to regulate their eating through bodily feedback: they eat when they are hungry and stop eating when they are full. In contrast, the *boundary model* proposes that restrained eaters regulate their eating to a self-imposed limit on their daily calorie intake (Herman & Polivy, 2008). Chronic dieters regulate their eating according to diet rules of permissible daily calorie intake. In many cases, these dieting rules reflect the dietary recommendations of the currently fashionable diet. These rules are used to guide food intake to achieve or maintain desirable weight.

Because regulation via dieting rules and calorie limits requires cognitive resources, it is liable to break down whenever dieters are unable or unwilling to invest cognitive resources in their eating attempts. Factors that interfere with cognitive control are therefore assumed to impair the regulation of food intake in dieters. Two sets of factors that tend to impair dieters' ability and motivation to control their eating are emotional distress and actual or perceived dietary violations. As long as this boundary is not broken, the restrained eater succeeds in restricting food intake. Once the diet is ruined, they tend to overeat[13]—if they eat "forbidden" foods, their dieting is ruined. For example, after eating the preload, restrained eaters have disinhibitory thoughts, like "I've already blown my diet, I might as well continue to eat," and start overeating. This motivational explanation of overeating has been termed the "what-the-hell-effect."[14] When they expect they will eat disallowed food later on, they start overeating the entire day.[15] The prospect of future overeating induces feelings of hopeless about the one's ability to adhere to personal rules of dietary restraint. In contrast, unrestrained eaters tend to display normal regulation of their eating behavior; after eating a preload (milkshake), they would eat less ice cream afterward.

For dieters who tend to think in a rigid, all-or-nothing fashion (Polivy & Herman, 1999), dieting may cause overeating. When dieters force themselves to ignore or override internal demands in their attempt to reduce

---

[13]The counterregulation behavior can also be modeled as game theory among successive selves within an individual. If you see yourself violate your diet today, you reduce your expectation that your diet will succeed. By this logic, an individual has incentives to develop self-enforcing cooperative arrangement with her future selves.

[14]Polivy and Herman (1985) coined the "what-the-hell" effect to describe the behavior of restrained eaters who overindulge when they exceed their daily calorie goal because they consider that the day is lost.

[15]However, dieters who are told that the milkshake preload contains few calories do not subsequently overeat. Moreover, those dieters whose diets were still intact showed greater activity in cognitive control regions.

their food intake, insensitivity to internal hunger cues and an over-reliance on external cues is likely to develop. To regulate their eating, they will have to rely more on calorie counting instead of internal hunger and satiety cues. One way to modify this "faulty" thought process is for dieters to avoid the division of calorie intake into daily units, and if diet goals have been violated on a given day, additional violation would not really matter. So, dieters need to recognize that every calorie ingested counts because it will contribute to fat stores or have to be worked off in some way.

Alcohol Myopia

Intoxication is another factor that disinhibits eating in dieters, known as *alcohol myopia*. Alcohol disarms willpower. Alcohol reduces self-awareness, thereby impairing one's ability to monitor one's behavior and contributing to failure at self-regulation. Indeed, people sometimes consume alcohol and other drugs to give themselves an excuse to lose self-control. Furthermore, alcohol tends to stimulate appetite—the intake of salty and fatty foods. In one study, subjects consumed 9% to 17% more calories after a single drink; a disproportionate number of them came from potato chips (Caton, Ball, Ahern, & Hetherington, 2004).

Social Influence

Social contexts influence our eating behavior.[16] Our tendency to conform can lead to overeating.[17] Herman, Roth, and Polivy (2003) showed that subjects ate fewer cookies when in the presence of a noneating observer than when alone. Roth (1999) explains observed behavior as the result of two social norms—one in favor of minimal eating and one in favor of matching the food intake of the other—ultimately driven by a concern for impression management. For instance, couples and families tend to be of similar sizes. If there is a majority of overweight people in a family, the frequency, quantity, and time spent eating puts more pressure on a person who is trying to lose weight. Studies (Stroebe, 2008) have confirmed that many people (especially women) eat less on dates or in other situations

[16]Evidence shows that young women tend to choose lower-calorie meals when dining with males than when eating with other women. The men's food choices remained consistent whether they ate with women or other men. The behavior reflects the women perception that smaller portions of food as more feminine and eating less will make them more attractive to men.
[17]Although this may be seen as a failure of self-control, people often make interpersonal acceptable a priority to their personal well-being.

where people can see them than when they are alone. When we are with others, we tend to mimic the speed at which they eat and how much they eat. The average amount others eat suggests the amount that is appropriate for us to eat. Likewise with portion size: we eat more when the portion size is increased. People are generally uncertain as to how much to eat on a given occasion and therefore rely on normative (appropriateness) cues as guides.[18] Thus, weight can be inherited, but it can be contagious.[19]

THE GOAL CONFLICT THEORY OF EATING BEHAVIOR

The *goal conflict theory of eating behavior* offers another perspective for why dieters often fail in their attempts to control their weight. Goals are mentally represented as desirable future states that the individual wants to attain. Stroebe et al. (2008) conceptualize the dilemma of dieters as a conflict between the goals of eating enjoyment and the goal of weight control. Chronic dieters want to reduce or at least maintain their present weight. At the same time, eating palatable food is a highly desirable goal for restrained eaters. Therefore, in order to succeed in their pursuit of the weight control goal, dieters have to shield the goal of weight control by inhibiting or devaluing the goal of eating enjoyment.

Weight control is normally the dominant goal for chronic dieters, who can operate for a long time without ever thinking about eating enjoyment. However, the environment is rich in stimuli signaling palatable food, and chronic dieters are sensitive to such temptation. For example, the palatable food cues, and even the approach of dinner time, are likely to reduce the motivation to control food intake. To the extent that the stimulus context increases the accessibility of the goal of enjoying palatable food, the goal of eating enjoyment might interfere with the goal of weight control. Thus, the smell or sight of palatable food is likely to activate thoughts about eating enjoyment in dieters.[20] In contrast, health primes activates goal of weight control and also feeling guilt (Okada, 2005).

Why do palatable food items have a more positive incentive value for restrained than for unrestrained eaters? One explanation is the differences in attitudes toward food. The exposure to external food cues, such

---

[18]Zajonc (1965) reviews research that shows that rats, chickens, and puppies eat significantly more when coupled with other hungry individuals. An apparently fully sated chicken, he reports, will eat up to two thirds as much again when introduced to a hungry companion chicken.

[19]Wansink (2006) reports that, on average, those who eat with one other person eat about 35% more than they do when they are alone; member of a group of four eats about 75% more; those in group of seven or more eat 96% more.

[20]Goals can be activated (primed) outside of awareness by exposing individuals to situational cues that in the past were frequently associated with the pursuit of a goal.

as high palatable foods, has a powerful effect on dieters. Exposure to palatable food cues elicits in restrained eaters pleasure-oriented, hedonic thoughts about food (attentional bias for short-term rewards), which then guide their behavior and lead to overeating, despite their chronic dieting goal (Papies et al., 2007). Restrained eaters are more likely than unrestrained eaters to access "hot" representations of palatable food stimuli, reflecting the arousing, consummatory features of the food (i.e., its taste and texture), whereas unrestrained eaters use "cool," informational representations of food items. This could lead to overeating on palatable, high-calorie foods, and eventually weight gain.[21] Fedoroff, Polivy, and Herman (1997) found that the smell of cookies baking increased cookie craving and cookie consumption for all participants (though more so for chronically dieting restrained eaters). Food cues thus appear to be an important influence on eating, and exposure to tasty food cues can undermine dieters' motivation to sustain their diet.

The goal conflict model suggests that a cognitive bias, known as *compensatory intentions*, influences dieters' decision to indulge. Compensatory intentions are formed as a means of relieving the discomfort of having indulged. Temptations elicit compensatory intentions.[22] Dieters who are tempted form compensatory intentions in an effort to balance the conflict of wanting to indulge and wanting to remain on their weight-loss diets. For example, people who have the goal to lose weight but also the desire to eat sweets may form the intention, "I'll eat this cookie now, but I will cut back later." However, evidence shows that dieters fail to follow through with their plan to compensate (Kronick & Knauper, 2010). Thus, these beliefs are detrimental if they are not implemented. Since these beliefs are formed under emotional circumstances, later on dieters may not be highly motivated or emotionally charged to follow through.

DIET AS A RISK FACTOR FOR WEIGHT GAIN

Does dieting ultimately result in weight loss or does it actually promote disordered eating patterns (such as binge eating) and eventually result in weight gain? Restraint theory suggests that an overreliance on cognitive

---

[21]Since it is difficult to enjoy one's food while thinking about one's weight, all plans about dieting and calorie restriction may be momentarily "forgotten." By the time these dieting thoughts are allowed to resurface, a dieter might decide to finish the meal with a sweet course, because the diet for the day will have been ruined anyway ("what-the-hell" cognitions).

[22]Compensatory behavior is similar to "Flex Points" Weight Watcher. Dieters are invited to use the "Flex Point" in "splurge contexts" in order to make eating out not only possible, but enjoyable.

control over eating, rather than physiological cues, may leave dieters vulnerable to overeating when these cognitive controls are disrupted by emotions or the intake of forbidden food (Herman & Polivy, 1980). The cognitive regulation of eating behavior is a controlled process that requires willpower (cognitive resources). If restrained eaters are able and motivated to concentrate on the regulation of their eating, they are quite capable of keeping to their diet rules. However, if their motivation or ability to regulate their eating is impaired, overeating will occur (i.e., the experience of strong emotions and a previous violation of the diet boundary).

It is also possible that individuals with a chronic overeating tendency may attempt to restrict their intake but ultimately fail in these efforts and show weight gain. Behavioral and physiological data suggest that restrained eating may be a proxy risk factor for vulnerability to weight gain. Lowe and Kral (2006) suggest that in certain predisposed individuals, restraint is primarily a result of a vulnerability to overeating. For example, restraint eaters tend to have lower resting metabolic rates, increased levels of fasting plasma triglycerides, reduced levels of leptin, and reduced fasting insulin levels. These characteristics would favor the storage of fat in restrained relative to unrestrained eaters, a tendency that would favor greater weight gain over time in restrained eaters. Stice et al. (2010) found that bulimic behavior predicted future increases in restraint, but restraint did not predict future increases in bulimic behavior. In short, it is possible that the dieters who restrict energy intake may be those who recognize that they are gaining weight and restrict energy intake as a protective strategy, so the weight problem may be the cause rather than the result of the restriction.

Furthermore, repeated or chronic food deprivation can sensitize food reinforcer effects, which may increase the reinforcing value of food over time. *Sensitization* is a term often used to define increases in drug reinforcement for the same drug dose over time. Several studies have shown that girls and adolescents who self-reported dieting are heavier later (Stice et al., 2010). If dietary restraint does involve intermittent periods of brief food deprivation, or deprivation of specific foods, these dieters may paradoxically be increasing the reinforcing value of these foods.

AWARENESS OF SELF-CONTROL ISSUES

Being aware of self-control problems can mitigate them. O'Donoghue and Rabin (1999) make a distinction between sophistication versus naivete. A sophisticated individual realizes that he or she will betray himself or herself in the future and thus undertakes actions now to restrict future behavior. A naïve individual is fully unaware of her future self-control problems and therefore prone to (wrongly) predict that she will "behave herself" in the future. This suggests that sophistication might help when we want to quit overeating. Sophisticated diners know that once faced with temptation, they will succumb. They will be reluctant to go to a restaurant, even one that offers a healthy menu, unless they believe it will help them to achieve the goals they have set while they were in their "right mind." In contrast, naïve diners believe (incorrectly) that they will eat healthy food and therefore may plan to behave one way but in fact behave differently. A naïve person may repeatedly delay quitting overeating, believing she will quit tomorrow, and this could lead to significant harms.

Naivete about future self-control problems can generate harm because the person fails to engage in such "self-management." Sophistication is "good" because it helps overcome self-control problems. Although the harm generated by individual decisions to indulge might be small, the accumulated harm generated by many decisions to indulge can be quite large. For example, cutting only 100 calories a day from our diets would prevent weight gain in most of the U.S. population (Hill & Peters, 1998). In short, the marginal impact of each decision occasion is negligible, as the consequences of these decisions only manifest themselves in aggregate. As a result, people are often blind to the cumulative effect.

Sophisticated individuals who understand their self-control problem take steps to combat it. They are able to recognize the situations in which they are likely to indulge and make "commitments" that help prevent this indulgence. They might, for instance, alter a situation in a way that will reduce the likelihood of indulging—for example by making sure to have only healthy desserts in the house—or they might choose to avoid the situation altogether—for example having no desserts in the house.

CONCLUSION

This chapter explains why diet preferences often vary from moment to moment by focusing on ways in which decision can be impaired. The long-term maintenance of a healthy lifestyle requires paying attention to why health preferences often change from moment to moment (Just, Mancino, & Wansink, 2007). Knowledge of factors that trigger overeating is of use to dieters and may lead to the development of beneficial weight loss strategies. Commitment devices, such as allowing individuals to preselect more healthful foods, may be an effective way to help individuals make food choices that align with their own future health goals. Findings from the National Weight Control Registry of those able to lose at least 30 lb and keep it off for a year suggest six key strategies for long-term success at weight loss maintenance: (1) daily physical activity, about one hour; (2) eating small portions; (3) eating regularly, especially breakfast; (4) regularly self-monitoring weight; (5) maintaining consistent eating throughout the year; (6) catching lapses before they turn into larger weight regains.[23] If a substantial number of individuals follow these strategies, it would have a significant public health effect. In sum, identifying factors that undermine successful maintenance of weight loss may aid health professionals in developing approaches to help dieters to maintain weight loss.

----

[23]The challenge of maintaining weight loss is shown by study of the Weight Watchers (WW) program (Stanley Heshka et al., 2003). People on WW were able, on average, to lose 12 lb after 6 months. But by the end of 2 years, almost half of the weight was regained. A major issue with losing weight quickly is that dieters do not learn much about how to sustain weight loss. By losing weight more slowly, however, people gain a better idea of what they need to do in the long term.

11

Self-Control Strategies

INTRODUCTION

How do individuals manage to pursue their long-term goals when they are constantly confronted with the allure of short-term alternatives? The problem of self-control will be present to some degree in all consumer decisions that involve a perceived conflict between the short-term and long-term outcomes of an action. For example, a dieter may mostly want to maintain his or her diet, but under some circumstances that motivation may diminish, and the dieter may knowingly violate the diet simply because at that moment he ceases to care much about losing weight. Self-control requires ignoring the attraction of short-term temptations in order to pursue other long-term goals. Such temptations are triggered by situational cues that promise immediate gratification at the cost of significant long-term rewards. Strong self-control is a very good predictor of later success in a wide range of academic and social issues. A huge body of research has linked good self-control to a broad range of desirable outcomes, including better mental health, more effective coping skills, healthier interpersonal relationships, superior academic performance, as well as less susceptibility to eating disorders and addiction (Offer, 2006).

This chapter provides an introduction to some basic principles of self-control, the reasons why people might want to precommit themselves to a goal, and of the devices they have at their disposal. While some people may be naturally more resistant to temptation, people can also train themselves to protect their long-term interests against temporary distractions.

THE SECRET OF SUCCESS: PRACTICE

The literature on great performers takes some of the magic out of great achievement. They show that talent is overrated and top performers spend hours rigorously practicing their craft[1]. There is no doubt that

---

[1] The same can be said about change in personality trait, regardless of one's temperamental endowment. The plasticity of the brain allows one to establish new attitude through years of practice, or to unlearn a bad habit, such as learned helplessness.

genes place a limit on our capacities. But the brain is also plastic. We mold our brain through what we do. Skill development depends on how repetition is organized.

Research shows that it takes approximately 10 years of intense work to acquire the level of expertise to thrive in any field (Gladwell, 2008). It also takes the brain 10,000 hours to assimilate all that it needs to achieve true mastery. The 10,000 hours rule translates into practicing 3 hours a day for 10 years, which is indeed a common training span for young people in sports. Success is the result of accumulative advantages.[2] This suggests that success is not so much ability as attitude. Success is a function of persistence and willingness to work hard. It is hard to achieve any difficult goal, or to carry out any long-range plan, unless you can make yourself persist at it. Many achievers regard their ability to function in spite of pain, rejection, or adversity to be among their outstanding accomplishment.

In his book *Outliers*, Malcolm Gladwell (2008) demonstrates that successful people are those who have been given opportunities and who have had the strength and presence of mind to seize them. Virtually every success story covered in the book involves someone or some group who work harder than their peers.[3] Similarly, Matthew Syed (2010) in his book *Bounce* shows that top performers excel not because of innate ability but because of dedicated practice. Success in most fields is not a reflection of innate skill, but rather a devoted and purposeful effort. In short, these authors conclude that while dedicated practice may not make one the best, it does maximizes one's personal potential.

SUCCESS AND SELF-CONTROL

Self-control is defined as the deliberate and conscious control of powerful impulses and desires, at the time they occur.[4] For example, it is the willpower that a bored student mobilizes to remain awake and concentrate.

---

[2]In human development, Martha Nussbaum and Amartya Sen thus prefer the word *capability* to *ability*. Different sorts of environments stimulate or fail to stimulate individuals to develop capability.

[3]For example, Bill Gates as a young computer programmer from Seattle attended high school that happened to have a computer club when almost no other high schools did. He then took advantage of the opportunity to use the computers at the University of Washington for hours. By the time he turned 20, he had spent well more than 10,000 hours as a programmer.

[4]Other terms for self-control include "self-binding," "pre-commitment," "commitment," "self-commitment," "self-regulation," and "constraint theory." Resolution, a related term, is defined as involving an intention to engage in certain action or stand firm against future temptation (Holton, 2009).

Self-control is measured by the ability to delay gratification in situations of intense temptation or stress.

A self-control problem represents an internal conflict between the pursuits of different goals, one of which is of greater long-term importance than the other. This conflict can lead to misbehavior—behaving differently from what one would have preferred if asked from a prior perspective.[5] For example, addiction, obesity, debt or bankruptcy, violence, unwanted pregnancy, school failures, anger, and so on, all colored by temptation and impulsiveness. In these decisions, the individual may seek short-term gains but long-term costs, given the eventual costs exceeding the benefit.

The essence of self-control (or intrapersonal conflict) is that people sometimes report feeling as though there were two selves inside them (Thaler & Shefrin, 1981). These two selves, one more present-oriented and the other more future-oriented, are battling for control. One self is a planner who is interested in the individual's long-run well-being; the other is a doer who is only concerned with short-run payoffs. In the context of the Dual-Model theory (as discussed in Chapter 7), the Planner represents Reflective System, and the Doer represents the Affective System.[6] The Planner is trying to promote your long-term well-being but must cope with the feelings of the Doer who is exposed to the temptations. Since actions are taken by the Doer, the Planner restricts the set of alternatives in order to mitigate the Doer's willingness to satisfy immediate gratification at the expense of long-term well-being.

For example, when people are under the influence of emotions, they often act in ways that they will regret later. If they can anticipate this tendency, they can take precautions of the kind chosen by Ulysses, when he had his men tie him to the mast as they approached the island of the Sirens (Elster, 2001). Able to foresee this temporary change in his preferences, he came up with an effective commitment device to foreclose his options. Similarly, the public authorities may do so on behalf of people.[7] Examples include the empty-fridge strategy, or legislating or imposing delays on the purchase of firearms (Camerer, Loewenstein, & Rabin, 2003).

---

[5]The documentary movie about, the youngest fighter to win the W.B.C. heavyweight title, portrays a man who squandered his talent and good fortune. He started out as a street criminal in Brooklyn and was saved from juvenile detention by Mr. D'Amato and his associates, who disciplined his natural volatility and turned him into a fighter. But Mr. Tyson never learned to control his self-destructive instincts.

[6]In the previous chapter, we reviewed the two-system conception of decision making. Some parts of the brain are impulsive, and other parts are prepared to enable us to resist temptation. Sometimes the two parts of the brain can be in conflict—a kind of battle that one or the other is bound to lose. For the dieter, the sight and smell of pizza, or any palatable food, triggers strong cravings that lead to preference reversal.

[7]The Illinois "self-exclusion program" allows problem gamblers to voluntarily enroll in the program to ban themselves from receiving prizes over $600. The program provides a tool for individuals to strengthen their resolve (tying their hands).

FIGURE 11.1   Payoff Matrix in the Prisoner's Dilemma

	Cooperate	Cheat
Cooperate	6 m, 6 m	10 y, 0
Cheat	0, 10 y	5 y, 5 y

Figure 11.1 shows a model of how we control our behavior. In this model, a person in cold (self-control) mode plans to foreclose options, engage in cue management, or publicly commit to a deadline. These strategies may reduce the self-control problems (e.g., effort may be spent controlling anger in a given activity). The level of investment varies from person to person. Those who exhibit greater tendency to become angry will require an allocation of more energy and time to modify the behavior.

Emotion State

___| invest_____ | stimulus_____ | act_____ | end_____post-state___

THE KEY INGREDIENTS OF SELF-CONTROL

Self-control depends on several factors, including commitment to goals, motivation, self-efficacy, monitoring of the self and its behaviors, and willpower. These factors are all necessary for effective self-control, and a breakdown or problem with any one of them can undermine self-control (Vohs, Baumeister, & Loewenstein, 2007).

Commitment to Goals

The more specific the goal,[8] the better able people are to reach it. Specific goals (or breaking up your goals into smaller subgoals) allow for better monitoring of progression toward the goal. Having only one goal makes self-control more successful than when people have two or more conflicting goals.[9] Effective self-control also requires disengaging from goals when progress is too slow.[10] People who disengage from seemingly impossible

---

[8]So rather than setting a vague goal such as "I will get healthy," set one with specific commitment to a time and place, "I will go to the health club at 7:30 A.M. tomorrow." That will make you more likely to follow through. Also, it is easier to postpone vague or open-ended tasks with distant deadlines than focused and short-term projects. Therefore, dividing projects into smaller and more defined parts could be helpful.

[9]"Do one thing and do it well," as Plato's counseled. With too many options, we often are afraid of making the wrong choice, so we end up doing nothing.

[10]Charles Schultz, creator of the "Peanuts" cartoon series, once said that no problem is so formidable that you cannot walk away from it. Although perseverance can be an admirable trait and is essential for all success in life, when taken too far it becomes self-destructive. Thus, it is important to know when to abandon goals that cannot be achieved, as when to increase one's efforts.

goals are mentally healthier than those who stay entrapped. Dropping the frustrating goals allows one to avoid attempting the impossible and use one's limited effort and time more effectively. In short, a successful self-control requires that one's goal be kept firmly in focus and reserve the most careful decision resources for the choices that matter most.

Motivation

One has to be motivated and committed to reach the goal. The more you want the goal, the more likely you are willing to make the efforts and sacrifices required to achieve it. For example, most people believe that smoking cigarettes is bad for them, and many have quit smoking in order to improve their odds of avoiding lung cancer in later life, but others may not value that outcome. Thus, motivation is a function of expectations of future benefit.

Self-Efficacy

Motivation may be impacted by perceptions of the possibility (or difficulty) that the goal can be attained. Much of modern psychology has emphasized the importance of *self-efficacy* as a crucial ingredient in success (Bandura, 1997). Self-efficacy refers to an individual's sense of competence or ability in general or in particular domains. Higher self-efficacy, or confidence, enhances the individual's motivation and effort. People who believe that they can succeed are more likely to make the effort in the first place. Similarly, self-confidence is defined as a favorable or unfavorable attitude toward the self. Confidence in one's abilities generally enhances motivation, making it a valuable asset for individuals with imperfect self-control (Benabou & Tirole, 2002). The confident individual is more likely to persist in the face of obstacles.[11]

An unrealistic belief in one's ability is the essence of overconfidence.[12] Overconfident individuals fail to recognize their own deficiency and likely overinvest in courses of action that are likely to

---

[11]The idea that confidence enhances performance is illustrated as $(E \times A) \pm TD = B$, in which effort (E) times ability (A), plus or minus task difficulty (TD) equals the behavioral outcome (B). A higher self-confidence enhances the individual's motivation and effort (A). This formula explains the incentive to develop and maintain the individual's self-confidence (Benabou & Tirole, 2002). Of course, the relationship between self-confidence and achievement can be circular. You feel good about yourself, in part, because you have accomplished something well. On the other hand, it is hard to imagine people taking the first step without self-confidence.

[12]For example, the National Institutes of Health (NIH) recommends that dieters start with an initial goal of no more than 10% of starting weight.

fail. If one constantly fails in attainting a goal, then one might do well to abandon the unattainable goal[13] (and redirect efforts more profitably). However, we tend to be lousy at recognizing this. Thus, overconfident individuals may embark on ventures they would otherwise have avoided.

In the context of health behavior, high self-efficacy predicts successful weight loss, abstinence from cigarette smoking, and alcohol consumption (Coon, Pena, & Illich, 1998; Rothman, 2000). But, the initial success may foster overconfidence. Thus, overconfident clients completing their treatment for alcohol abuse are more likely to relapse (Goldbeck, Myatt, & Aitchison, 1997). People who successfully complete the initial phase of treatment tend to believe that they have proven that they can do it, but quitting may be easier than maintaining the changed behavior over the long run. As a 12-step treatment for addiction states: "every day brings you one day closer to your next relapse." The point of statement is to encourage addicts to minimize the threat of overconfidence that may develop later in recovery and remind them that addiction is a permanent condition, regardless of how long abstinence is maintained.

Self-Monitoring

Self-monitoring is central to self-control. Monitoring involves being aware of the self's behavior or responses and comparing them to a goal.[14] Monitoring allows people to assess distance to the goal. This can be done by looking back at how far one has come or how much more has to be done. Seeing how far one has come may be more effective in promoting self-control than how much more work is ahead (positive framing). Believing that one has come a long way increases commitment to the goal, thereby leading to heightened efforts to reach it.[15]

---

[13]For example, if I were to try to break into the world of modern dance, after the first few rejections the logical response might be practice even more. But after the 10,000th rejection, maybe I should realize this is not a viable career option.

[14]A key success factor to weight-loss maintenance is the use of self-monitoring (Wing & Phelan, 2005). Successful dieters count calories and otherwise carefully monitor their food intake, and the cessation of monitoring often undermines dietary efforts. Self-monitoring includes weighing frequently, recoding food intake, and physical activity. For example, evidence shows that people who wear pedometers get more exercise, lose weight, and lower their blood pressure. For many, a pedometer provides motivation, accountability, and a sense of control.

[15]Show that focusing on the unaccomplished portion of a goal provides bigger incentives for those who have a deeper commitment to the goal, while focusing on the accomplished portion better motivates people whose commitment is more uncertain.

Willpower

Willpower is another important ingredient in self-control. Sticking to one's plan is hard work. Without the willpower to bring about changes, the best laid plans and all the monitoring in the world will not be good enough. Willpower represents vitality or psychological energy that one uses to resist other temptations in order to work toward one's goal. When in vital states, people are more active and productive, and they cope better with stress and challenges. Self-control is governed by a limited mental resource. Engaging in one self-control task leaves less energy available for subsequent self-control tasks (Baumeister, Muraven, & Tice, 2000). For example, diets are more frequently abandoned in evenings more than mornings (Vohs & Faber, 2007), which suggest that as the day wears on willpower gets depleted. Certain states of mind undermine self-control. For example, reformed alcoholics are far more likely to relapse if they are depressed, anxious, or tired (Elster, 1999).[16] Rest appears to be the most common route to replenishment, such that when people get a good sleep their self-control is better.

Summary

In sum, if you want to know whether someone will stick to a given resolution, you'll need to know how realistic or specific the resolution is, about her motivation to abide by the resolution, the strength of her desire, her level of confidence, and the strength of her willpower, and so on. Thus, one's action is determined not only by the strength of one's desire and one's determination but also by one's willpower, and the latter component is affected by repeated exercise.

SELF-CONTROL STRATEGIES

Self-control strategies help a person to commit to behave in a certain way in the future, even though he or she may wish to behave otherwise when the time comes. The following sections describe an array of self-control strategies people use to protect themselves against temptations to maintain long-term goals, despite the short-term costs. The discomfort often associated with dieting or physical exercise is a price people have to pay to attain their long-term health goals.

External commitment strategies are often used for avoiding sources of temptation, or asking for controls. *Cognitive strategies* involve changing

---

[16]As noted before, the depletion of willpower is the same as leaving the person with System 1 (unconscious, fast, but inflexible system).

one's thoughts or beliefs about a particular behavior, such as self-deception (strategic ignorance) about the costs and benefits of perseverance or indulgence. *Personal rules* include rules such as a resolution to smoke only after meals, jog twice a week, always finish what you started, and many similar "promises to oneself." *Automatic self-control* may occur in the absence of conscious intent and even without the person being aware that they are engaging in goal-directed behavior. When an action becomes automatic the need for willpower disappears.

EXTERNAL COMMITMENT STRATEGIES

External commitment devices are used to substitute for individual's deficient willpower to avoid sources of temptation. It is better to engineer the decision context so that it is impossible to succumb to a weakness of will than to rely on one's ability to resist temptation. External strategies involve avoiding the occasions that trigger the desire to consume. For example, people who want to quit smoking often learn that they must stop drinking as well, because alcohol serves as a cue for cigarette craving and also causes disinhibition. It is also recommended people who want to stop drinking or smoking avoid places where these activities go on.

Social policies may reduce the cues that influence consumption. In the case of smoking, the government has assisted in removing cues to smoke, including smoking bans in public places and bans on smoking advertisements. Ultimately, cue management is used to facilitates cue extinction or deconditioning craving (eliminating positive responses to unhealthy behaviors). Cue extinction involves repeated exposure to stimuli associated previously with drug use without using the drug in an attempt to extinguish an addict's conditioned responses to such cues.

Precommitment Strategies

This strategy allows a person who foresees being tempted by a particular stimulus in the future to take measures in the present that will prevent him or her from giving in to the temptation. Precommitment might take the form of fully eliminating the alternative that is currently unwanted but apt to be preferred by one's future self. By precommitment, an individual might limit his/her freedom of action. For example, addicts make efforts to keep temptation at a distance or out of sight. One may adopt the practice of having no alcoholic beverages at home so that one has to go a store to buy them. An addict may eliminate the option for drug use (at least in the short run) by checking-in to a remote treatment facility.

Pharmacologic agents such as naltrexone and buprenorphine reduce the high available from some substances. In sum, these strategies take the form of actions that can be expected to make the currently unwanted alternative less desirable.

Similarly, individuals may eliminate options by making the choice of the early, smaller reward physically impossible.[17] For example, an individual may place his or her alarm clock across the room to foreclose options upon which he or she might focus during hot visceral states (going back to sleep), or leaving his or her credit card at home to avoid impulse purchases of tempting goods. Parents may use this strategy to discourage youths' sedentary behaviors, by making sedentary alternatives less rewarding. For example, locating video game systems in an unheated, unfinished basement may reduce video game playing.[18]

People attempt to control their consumption of "tempting" foods by purchasing small packages, even when the unit price is lower for larger packages. Regular smokers sometimes buy cigarettes by the pack, even though it would be cheaper and more convenient to buy cartons. Wertenbroch (1998) showed that consumers with a need for self-control prefer to buy vice products in smaller quantities than comparable virtue products, thus rationing their vice consumption. Importantly, these consumers forgo quantity discounts for the vice products, paying a small-size premium that can be conceived of as a self-control premium.[19]

In an experimental study, Downs et al. (2009) examined consumer choice by manipulating selections of food items. The researchers increased the convenience of healthful sandwich options and imposed a tiny immediate cost for selecting a sandwich off the menu. The results showed that consumers who received the healthful featured menu were more likely to choose low-calorie sandwiches when it was more convenient to do so. In short, these studies demonstrate that a simple nudge produced behavior change.[20]

---

[17]Schelling (1984) cited an anecdote illustrating this strategy. When George Steiner first visited Georg Lukacs, he was overwhelmed by the volume of Lukacs work. When he asked how he could accomplish so much, Lukacs replied "House arrest, Steiner, house arrest."

[18]For another example, consider the case of tax withholding. About 75% of Americans get refunds when they file their tax returns, with average refund about of $2000. These refunds are like interest-free loans to the government. Although taxpayers could adjust their withholding rates to reduce the size of their refund and earn more interest on these funds, many prefer to get the refund as a way of being forced to save. When the refund comes, it feels like a windfall.

[19]This also translates into a smaller price elasticity of demand for vices than for virtues.

[20]Observed that reducing the size of trash bins brought about a dramatic decrease in garbage production. When it was more difficult to dispose of garbage, consumers became more careful about the amount of waste they generated.

Imposing Costs

This strategy involves the voluntary attachment of a monetary fine for failure to act according to long-term preferences.[21] For example, joining a health club is the penalty of monetary loss if one fails to show up regularly ("I paid $600. I better use it").[22] One may be required to pay a relatively large cancellation fee for missing a medical test. Some former alcoholics take disulfiram (Antabuse), a drug that has the effect of making the user violently ill if he or she takes a drink. The drug helps people avoid drinking for about a week. Like Antabuse users, individuals who have the gastric bypass procedure (stomach stapling) drastically reduce their capacity to overeat. On the average, the procedure reduces the stomach pouch from a quart to a less than an ounce (Steele et al., 2009).[23]

In the context of weight loss, evidence (Ayers, 2010) shows that people who have financial incentives to lose weight are much more successful at dieting than those who do not. By making the future reward relevant to the present, financial incentives counter present bias behavior. Volpp et al. (2008) showed that the amount of weight loss depended on whether people staked small, daily amounts of their own money toward their goal. The researchers encouraged the deposits by matching what participants invested. The money would be lost if the monthly weight target was not reached. After 16 weeks, the group that put up its own money lost an average 14 lb (toward a 16-pound goal) and earned $378 each, and the control group with no incentives lost just 3.9 lb each. The study demonstrates the powerful motivation of *loss aversion*. The concept of loss aversion implies that losses loom larger than gains (about twice as large). When it comes to incentives, people hate giving up something they already own. They work twice as hard to avoid the loss than to secure a reward of equal amount.

---

[21]Thaler et al (2008) cites a scenario in which he used a similar strategy to help a new junior faculty member to complete his doctoral thesis. He made a deal with the faculty member that he would write a series of checks for $100, payable on the first day of each of the next few months. Thaler would cash each check if the new faculty member did not deliver a copy of a new chapter of his thesis by certain time. Thaler promised to use the money to have a party to which the new faculty member would not be invited. The strategy worked. The faculty member finished on time and no check was cashed.

[22]This strategy explains why individuals choose relatively more expensive annual gym memberships over "pay as you go" options, even though the latter would be less expensive for most users (DellaVigna & Malmendier, 2006).

[23]The over-the-counter Alli (orlistat) is a popular weight-loss drug (orlistat is available with a prescription), partially blocks the body's ability to absorb fat. Like the Antabuse, the users who eat too much fat immediately experience the unpleasant side effects, such as gas, diarrhea, and abdominal pain.

A great example of imposing costs in weight-reduction programs is demonstrated by Albert Ellis (2005), the creator of Rational-Emotive Therapy. He discussed the case of a Jewish woman who had inadequate control over an obsessive behavior. Although she wanted to stop the behavior and promised repeatedly to desist, the woman seemed not to be able to resist doing it at certain times. Dr. Ellis had the woman give him a large amount of money in order to implement the following plan. Whenever the woman manifested an instance of the forbidden obsessive behavior, Dr. Ellis would send $50 of her money to the American Nazi Party. The patient gained control over the behavior.[24] Perhaps the awareness that breaking your diet will contribute to a cause that you do not approve will help you resist that slice of chocolate cake.

At a policy level, there is a large body of literature indicating that increasing prices or taxes on unhealthy activities is an effective means of changing behavior.[25] Policies to increase tobacco taxes appear to have substantial benefits in discouraging smoking activities. Similarly, evidence on the effect of alcohol prices on consumption suggests that adolescents are price responsive and some studies have found that both alcohol participation and binge drinking are responsive to alcohol prices (Saffer & Dave, 2006).

Reward Strategy

This strategy involves setting up rewards contingent on choosing the delayed reward. As a self-imposed incentive, people reward themselves for pursuing long-term goals (e.g., receiving a reward for losing weight). Reward changes the choice situation and nudges the individual to act according to long-term goals. The reward strategy brings forward the benefits of undertaking desirable activities (from a health perspective) or of avoiding undesirable ones. Increasingly, health insurance systems are incentivizing health choices via reduced premiums and cash payments. For example, rewards for health-related behavior are a key feature of German health insurance systems.[26] Individuals are offered bonuses for

---

[24]Web sites such as StickK.com motivate people to make changes in their lives by signing contracts: if they fail in their goals, it costs them money.

[25]When West Virginia revoked driving permits for students who were under the age of 18 and who dropped out of school, the dropout rate fell by one-third in the first year. While teens tend to be oblivious to the long-term benefits of getting a high school diploma, they do appreciate the short-term punishment of losing a license.

[26]Providing reward for reducing unhealthy behaviors is a practice that most parents do with their children by offering them rewards of various kinds (usually money) if they do not take up smoking before a certain age.

participating in check-up programs, dieting, and smoking cessation. The bonuses usually take the form of reductions in copayments (Schmidt, 2008). However, some may raise moral concern that we are bribing people to do some things that after all are in their own interest to do so. Positive financial incentives to eliminate bad behaviors could also lead to the problem of moral hazard. That is, people might be actively encouraged to engage in unhealthy behavior in the expectation of getting some kind of reward if they then give up or reduce the behavior concerned. However, monitoring or checking this kind of reaction might be difficult.[27]

Default Option (Status Quo)

Thaler and Sunstein (2008) build on the fact established by behavioral economics that "defaults" and "starting points" matter. So, for instance, if workers are automatically enrolled in a pension plan, but with the freedom to opt out if they wish, most stay in. But if they are not automatically enrolled, but have to make a conscious decision to opt in, then most stay out. The use of default in retirement savings is one clear example. The save-more-tomorrow plan allows employees to commit to saving in the future by taking the contributions out of future pay increases rather than current income, as well as by contributing the default. Initial applications have shown widespread adoption (by 78% of those who are offered participation, with 80% of them remaining in the program through four pay raises). The same observation applies to organ donation. In the case of organ donation, if the "default" is one where permission is assumed to be automatically given, unless one is carrying a card denying permission. The policy has resulted in increase in organs available for transplants (Johnson & Goldstein, 2003). Thus, significantly more people are willing to be donors when the default is to be a donor than when an active choice must be made to be a donor.

In the context of food, this bias can be exploited by making the healthiest choice, the one that follows the path of least resistance. For example, fast food restaurants that now offer soda as the default choice with a combo meal can instead make a bottle of water the default option,

---

[27]Consider, for example, the experience of New York City schools with a program that pays students for improving their standardized tests scores. Initial results have been extremely encouraging. Many psychologists warn against extrinsic rewards. They argue that external rewards can undermine the joy of learning for its own sake. For example, Edward L. Deci argues that once reward systems are over, students will choose not to do the activity. Economists, on the other hand, argue that with students who are failing, everything should be tried, including rewards. While students may be simply attracted by financial incentives at first, later on it could foster a love of learning.

with soda being a substitution available only on request. In short, the shift in thinking is the result of reframing the default option (choice context), which nudges people toward good decisions while they have the right to make bad ones. Defaults are sticky—people stay in them.

COGNITIVE STRATEGIES

Cognitive strategies involve changing one's thoughts or beliefs about a particular behavior. Cognitive strategies help us to find a way to make the situation work for us. We may not be able to control the external environment, but we control how we think about it.

Mental Representation of Goal and Reward

This strategy relates to our ability to access to cold cognition (e.g., focus on the negative side of the chocolate cake—calories). A good example of this strategy is the research on delay of gratification by Metcalfe and Mischel (1999). In the study, children were better able to delay gratification when actively reinterpreting a tempting food in a manner designed to reduce its affective qualities (e.g., likening marshmallows to clouds) or distracting themselves by thinking about something else. The transformation of hot and motivating representations ("it looks yummy") into cool ones ("it looks like a cloud") facilitates willpower in the delay of gratification. When attention is not focused on the tempting reward stimuli, it makes sustained delay of gratification less effortful. In short, the crucial skill is the way they allocated their attention. Instead of getting obsessed with the "hot stimulus," the children distracted themselves by avoiding thinking about the marshmallow. This "out of sight, out of mind" strategy can increase our resolve.[28]

Creating Delays (Cooling-off Period)

The goal of this strategy is to put more time between the choice and the ability to act upon it. By doing so, we will not fall prey to basing decisions entirely on what happens to be in our mind in the immediate moment. The mere passage of time can lower the temperature of desire. Strong emotions often dissipate with time. We usually get into trouble when we act impulsively without thinking things through. In general, when people

---

[28]The follow-up studies of these children showed that those who were able to deal with hot emotions were also better able to delay gratification (e.g., they achieved higher academic success and savings for retirement).

contemplate any action for days or weeks they may choose differently. This is captured by the common advice to "sleep on" a decision. Cooling-off laws enacted at both the state and federal level allows consumers to return certain types of purchases within a few days of the transaction. Such laws can be viewed as devices for combating the effects of projection bias[29] and the salespersons' incentives to hype. Cooling-off periods that force consumers to reflect on their decisions for several days can decrease the likelihood that they end up owning products that they should not. In the context of food, eating fast may provide insufficient time for the full effect of satiety signals as food reaches the intestine to operate. Fast eating is a behavior that might have been learned in infancy and could be reversed, although this might not be easy. Thus, one way of increasing satiety is slowing down the consumption of food and concentrate on the perception of every bite, which is typically fast in the obese individuals (Otsuka et al., 2006). The evidence shows that trying to slow down mealtimes for children would have an impact on future obesity rates.

Fight Emotion with Emotion

This strategy involves cultivation of an emotion to forestall the development of a contrary one. Francis Bacon once remarked that "reason did not have its own force, but had to get its way by playing one passion against another." That is, reason has to acquire the same kind of power, the same motivation that passions have, if it is sometimes to overcome them.[30] Reason and passion must compete for control of the person's behavior using the same kind of currency. Thus, the individual may train himself to care less about certain desires, or even to find them repulsive, by associating them with vivid, disgusting images (e.g., associating fatty foods with images of clogged arteries) and conversely by pairing positive images with delayed-gratification actions (receiving an award, achieving success, etc.). For example, the alcoholic struggling to maintain abstinence may cultivate an emotional revulsion to activities that lead to drinking.[31]

---

[29]Projection bias occurs when people behave as if their future preferences will be more like their current preferences than they actually will be. Projection bias can cause misguided purchases of durable goods, such as home treadmills, stationary bikes, and other equipment that ends up gathering dust.

[30]Spinoza, a seventeenth century philosopher, recommended that we fight a negative emotion with an even stronger but positive emotion brought about by reasoning and intellectual effort. Central to his thinking was the notion that the subduing of the passions should be accomplished by reason-induced emotion and not just pure reason alone.

[31]Another strategy would be to think about how one would feel afterwards, if one would break one's diet. Research on condom use has shown that anticipated regret about having unsafe sex increased condom use.

Strategic Ignorance

People also attempt to reduce the intensity of temptation, the gap between their long- and short-run preferences, through strategic ignorance or self-deception about the costs and benefits of perseverance or indulgence (Benabou & Tirole, 2002; Carrillo & Mariotti, 2000). In many situations, people have the option to acquire information about the costs and benefits of their actions, but they do not.[32] For example, individuals with inaccurately exaggerated estimates of the risk of smoking may remain strategically ignorant of the true risk in order to increase their determination to avoid smoking.[33]

Mindfulness

The strategy refers the sense of being aware of what we are feeling and doing. If we are mindful of our emotions, we can make the following choice: Do we want to act upon the craving or anger, or do we simply want to observe it? Mindfulness training invites the individual first to label internal sensations and cognitive preoccupation as an urge and to foster an attitude of detachment from the urge. The goal is to identify and accept the urge but not act on the urge or attempt to fight it. The technique invites the individual to observe and accept any negative thought as an event that occurs in the mind rather than as an absolute truth.

In the context of obesity and addiction, mindfulness might mean becoming aware of triggers for cravings and accepting the distress associated with those cravings. Patients learn how to "just be with, and feel" bad moods without turning to food or drugs (Kabat-Zinn, 1994). Learning to notice and accept thoughts about drugs may interrupt an automatic craving response by allowing for an attentional shift away from the craving response. This may be valuable for helping the impulsive individual to develop a greater awareness of their current emotional state, to bring into conscious control their behavioral tendency, and to allow for a more considered response.[34]

---

[32]If, for instance, a person is deciding whether to embark on a specific project, she has the option to get feedback from colleagues about the likely fruitfulness of that project. The rational thinking implies having more information allows people to make better decisions. However, strategic ignorance requires not acquiring information because doing so increases the likelihood of changing one's mind.

[33]Benjamin Franklin once said "Keep your eyes wide open before marriage, half shut afterwards".

[34]Cope Moyer (2006), a recovering addict writes: "I was born with a hole in my soul," and "a pain that came from the reality that I just wasn't good enough." Being mindful of his pain was a key in his recovery.

PERSONAL RULES

Personal rules (or internal commitments) are promises to cooperate with the individual's own subsequent motivational states (Ainslie, 2001). The basic idea for this strategy comes from turning individual choices into a matter of principle. The strategy requires perceiving a clear link between behavior today and behavior in the future, which transforms the impulsive act from an isolated decision into a pattern of behavior. For example, smoker can reason that if I break my resolution to give up smoking, I will not quit smoking for good. Personal rule as a self-control strategy helps people see current decisions as predictors of future behavior and the awareness of this linkage helps them overcome temptation.

Intrapersonal Dilemma (Multiple Selves)

As discussed in Chapter 6, time inconsistency (hyperbolic discounting) is an expression of a "divided self." Hyperbolic discounting predicts preference reversal. The individual who in the morning prefers to avoid overeating may be aware that this preference is in danger of being defeated by his or her future self in the evening. Further, this reversal of preference will lead to regret afterward. The conflict between current and future selves can be illustrated by the Prisoner's Dilemma. In the Prisoner's Dilemma, two accomplices are arrested and interrogated in separate rooms. The authorities give each prisoner the same choice: Confess your shared guilt (in effect, betray your partner) or remain silent (and be loyal to your partner). If one betrays and the other stays silent, the defector goes free, and the silent, loyal one spends 10 years in jail. If both remain loyal, both get 6 months. If both betray the other, both get 5 years. Each person has the temptation to cheat the other to gain lower punishment. When both players pursue their own self-interest, both do worse than they would have if somehow they could have jointly and credibly agreed that each would remain silent (Figure 11.1).

Likewise, the strategic action that can be taken by the present self to forestall an anticipated reversal of preference is to find a method to precommit (cooperate) to the currently desired alternative. For instance, an alcoholic who wants to quit might be willing to avoid drinking tonight if he thinks that he will not drink in the future, but not if he thinks that he will soon start again. Knowledge that he was able to overcome the desire to drink last night might make him more confident that he will be able to overcome the desire in the future, and thus more likely to resist tonight. Thus, a lapse damages self-credibility and causes failure. In short, if early selves resist temptation, future selves will be optimistic about their own ability to resist, but if early selves never overcome temptation, later selves will be more skeptical. But, if an addict knows in his heart he is going to use someday, why not today?

Bundling Choices (*"If Not Now, When?"*)

The understanding of the intrapersonal dilemma implies making a choice in a whole bundle (global approach). The decision to stop smoking is in effect a decision to begin a pattern of behavior. Not smoking tonight makes it easier not to smoke tomorrow and not smoking tomorrow makes it easier not to smoke the next day, and so on. The idea is that the individual should come to see each decision as a possible predictor of future ones, so that giving in today raises the probability that he will do the same in the future (Ainslie, 2001). By tying together sequences of choices, the individual aligns his short-term incentives with his long-run interests. The fear of creating precedents and losing faith in oneself then creates an incentive that helps counter the bias toward instant gratification.

Howard Rachlin (2000) argues that self-control comes from choosing "patterns" of behavior over time rather than individual "acts."[35] While the physical independence of today and tomorrow is real enough, the fact remains that actions today affect actions tomorrow. To smoke the cigarette tonight is to fail to perceive the connection between tonight's act and the pattern of acts over many nights and days. The patterns of choice motivate a person to be less impulsive. For example, if one's pattern of "a healthy breakfast" consists of juice, cereal, a bran muffin, and skim milk, then this person would not substitute apple pie for the bran muffin, because it would break up the pattern. Other examples include monthly savings targets, jogging twice a week, writing five pages a day, always finishing what one starts, conducting one's life with dignity, and many similar "promises to oneself."

For an addict, the recovery requires a measure of integration between his different selves and between his past and his present. Thus, it is not a good idea to make many sorts of decisions on a case-by-case basis (local choice). On a case-by-case basis, most of us would be having that second dessert or drinking that third martini at a party. Moreover, personal rules lower deliberative efforts (exerting willpower) that might otherwise be engaged by each specific instance of temptation.

Public Pledges

This strategy relies on the fact that humans care intensely about how they are perceived. When we make public pledges and then are reminded that we are not living up to those pledges, we effectively turn the people around us into our enforcers. We feel that the eyes of our friends and

---

[35]Warning! This mental trick may also account for "rigidity" as discussed below.

colleagues are on us and that they are degrading us. In short, self-reputation gives force to self-control. Social context matters and you are more likely to succeed if keeping your promise is a matter of honor.

AUTOMATIC SELF-CONTROL

The strategies discussed so far have considered self-control to be a conscious, active process. *Automatic self-control* strategies may occur in the absence of conscious intent (Gollwitzer & Sheeran, 2006). These strategies can make later self-control more automatic and therefore less reliant on willpower strength. They help to develop habits that reduce the demands on our cognition.

Implementation Strategy (If→Do Rules)

To maintain self-control (willpower) efforts when they are urgently needed, they have to be converted from conscious and effortful to automatic activation. The psychologist Peter Gollwitzer (1993) shows that by transforming goals into specific contingency plan, such as in the form "if X, then Y" (e.g., "if I see French fries, then I will avoid them"), we can markedly increase the chance of success. Such plans produce automatic behavior by intentionally delegating the control of one's goal-directed thoughts, feelings, and behaviors to specific situational cues. This means that the person does not have to exert deliberate effort when behavior is controlled by implementation intention strategy. As a result, the self should not become depleted. The self-control strategy creates a strong link between a situational cue (if-component) and a goal-directed response (then-component). For example, "if I start a project, then I will tell myself that I can complete this task." Research evidence supports that implementation intentions were associated with goal attainment in domains ranging from cancer screenings, diet, recycle, and physical exercise (Gollwitzer, Gawrilow, & Oettingen, 2010).

It is important to make distinction between goal intentions and implementation intentions. Typically, implementation intentions work in the service of goal intentions. Having just a goal intention is not enough. One will have to deliberate about how to implement it, and one may either forget to do so or simply decide to procrastinate. For example, in one study (Gollwitzer et al., 2010) a simple goal intention to perform a breast self-examination was acted upon by 50% of the subjects. However, the percentage increased to 100% by adding an implantation strategy about exactly when to do it.

Finally, implementation strategy is most effective when the specified plans address participants' key self-control problems. For instance, developing and implementing a plan to have a salad everyday for lunch may be beneficial, but it is unlikely to be an effective way to manage snacking while watching TV. Thus, if snacking at night is the primary problem, then the plan needs to address that challenge.

The Counteractive-Control Strategy

This strategy suggests that in the presence of temptation cues, individuals activate the overriding goals, which reminds them of their long-term priorities and helps them resist the temptations. For example, when fattening food is served, dieters activate the goal of dieting, which in turn enables them to avoid the forbidden foods. The idea complements the implementation strategy that the presence of an actual temptation in the environment may lead to an activation of the higher priority (long-term) goal. Thus, automatic goal activation may dominate situational control and promote the personal priorities (Fishbach, Friedman, & Kruglanski, 2003, 2006). Consequently, the mere presentation of a temptation-related cue in the environment (e.g., a delicious chocolate cake) automatically activates the planned behavior (e.g., a slim figure). For example, a study found that female dieters expressed greater body dissatisfaction when hungry. It seems that food deprivation serves as an "alert signal" that encourages self-control and successful implementation of dieting intentions among restrained eaters.

Unlike the resource-demanding self-control mechanisms, the activation of the automatic goal tends to be relatively independent of cognitive resources. Given our limited cognitive resources for conscious self-control, delegating control to situational cues is an effective way to bridge the gap that exists between our best intentions and the successful attainment of our goals.

THE HIDDEN COST OF SELF-CONTROL

How can self-control sometimes make us worse off? Many people have self-control problems of the opposite type, such as tightwads who cannot get themselves to spend enough, or workaholics[36] who cannot take a break. Both underregulation and overregulation are often just two sides

---

[36]One dictionary (Merriam-Webster) defines a workaholic as "a compulsive worker."

of the same coin.[37] For example, I may believe that I should take a vacation from my hectic life style, and I know that one week of vacation will not make any difference to my long-term success. But I just cannot convince myself to abstain from working. Excessive controlled appetites are as socially dysfunctional as those that are excessively uncontrolled. The miser is no more socially attractive than the profligate.

Ainslie (2001) argues that compulsive behaviors arise as side effects of successful attempts to alleviate the weakness of the will. Baumeister, Heatherton, and Tice (1994) observe that obsessions and compulsions are attempts to compensate for some self-control deficit. The rigid behavior occurs when an individual is so afraid of appearing weak to himself that every decision becomes a test of his willpower.[38] Such excessively rigid rules correspond well to compulsive or obsessive behaviors (e.g., the workaholic or the anorexic). Compulsions erode surprise, so that compulsive people are apt to get just as little long-range pleasure as impulsive ones. For them surprise is dangerous. The future ought to be known. Zabelina, Robinson, and Anicha (2007) showed individuals high in self-control were rated as less spontaneous compared with individuals low in self-control. Thus, there seems to be a trade-off in that self-control promotes consistency at the expense of spontaneity.

CONCLUSION

The ultimate goal of the study of behavioral economics is to help us overcome self-control problems, the lack of which contributes to a vast number of problems, including obesity. Self-control (or developing stronger willpower) is no simple skill, and many of us spend much of our lives seeking ways to make our minds "behave." The challenge is turning the self-control strategies into habits, which requires years of diligent practice to outsmart our desires. To be human is to fight a lifelong uphill battle for self-control. Moreover, individuals' exposure to short-term rewards does not occur in a social vacuum. Social organizations may provide external means of self-control, such as incentives, sanctions, and rules that

---

[37]Psychologists call this excessive foresight hyperopia. It is the opposite of myopia (nearsightedness). They are so obsessed with preparing for the future that they cannot enjoy the present, and they end up looking back sadly for missing out on life's pleasures. People tend to feel guilty about pleasures right afterwards, but as time passes, the guilt dissipates.

[38]The Movie Doubt (2008 release) details a conflict between the church's Father Flynn and the school's principal, Sister Aloysius. Although the movie raises philosophical questions about conservative versus progressive religious values, it is also about rigidity versus openness and suspicion and about how far one is willing to go to avoid one's doubt.

are designed to help individuals overcome temptations. Social control as substitute for self-control may reduce the demand for self-control efforts. Finally, learning self-control strategies can improve our well-being. Achieving well-being requires learning to exert self-control over our destructive impulses. Foregoing short-term temptations to pursue distal goals of longevity, fitness, thinness, education, wealth, and other options has enabled humans to make their lives happy and comfortable in ways most animals cannot even imagine.

12

Policy Implications and Conclusion

INTRODUCTION

In economics, the rational choice model is a starting point. Rational choice means that individuals understand their own preferences, make perfectly consistent choices over time, and try to maximize their own well-being. The rational choice implies choosing according to long-term outcomes rather than short-term ones. In this ideal world, self-control would never be a problem. We simply calculate the total values of our long-term goals and compare them with our immediate gratification and conclude that we are better off to resist the short-term temptation. By doing so, we would avoid overeating and weight gain.

At the basic level, obesity is the result of individual choices about diet and exercise. Rational food decisions often involve a trade-off between short-term gains of sensory pleasure and longer-term gains of health and wellness. In choosing food, people want to maximize their own utility (happiness). However, findings from behavioral economics research suggest that even when people are motivated to make healthy choices, external constraints in the decision process can prevent them from choosing optimally. People have self-control problems and they make self-defeating choices. Most of us prefer immediately gratifying short-term pleasure over our long-term goal of eating healthy. This book has offered several reasons for why people go astray when making food decisions. Errors in choices arise from systemic decision biases, emotion, and the limits of cognitive capacity.

More than 60% of Americans are considered either obese or overweight. Given the adverse effects obesity has on health, it is hard to claim that Americans are making ideal diet choices. At the same time, Americans spend in the aggregate many billions of dollars each year trying to lose weight through dieting or exercise, indicating our desire to slim down. There exists a gap between our declared intentions and actual behaviors. Therefore, people's current choices do not promote their well-being. If choices do not reveal an individual's true preferences, then the restriction of personal choice becomes justifiable.

CHOICE ARCHITECTURE

Insights from behavioral economics provide a more accurate understanding of the determinants of individual behavior. The behavioral economic framework explains why people appear so inconsistent when their behavior is viewed through the lens of the conventional rational model. We tend to pursue immediate gratification in ways that we ourselves do not appreciate in the long run. We are very committed to our long-term goal of eating healthy food, and yet, in the moment temptations arise that often trump up our long-term plan. Behavioral economics shows errors and biases in consumers' decision-making processes and questions the claim that people always make choices that are in their best interest. The goal of behavioral economics is to understand these decision errors and find ways for people to avoid temptation and exert self-control. By studying individuals' decision-making biases, behavioral economists suggest how to improve decisions and policy interventions that could help consumers avoid making problematic choices. These policy interventions can be seen as a form of libertarian paternalism that guides consumers to be better off without necessarily restricting their choices.

Many food policies that are designed to appeal to highly rational mind (e.g., fat taxes, detailed information labels) are likely to have little impact (Wansink, 2006). These policies assume that people's food-related behavior is a function of rational decision making. Although in limited cases, this may be true, but in most cases, marketing environments (i.e., packaging, price, and promotion) influence peoples' consumption decisions in ways that are anomalous to rational decision making. Thus, food policies need to account for decision biases. Significant improvements in reducing obesity and overweight may come from approaches that account not only for rational consumers but also for consumers whose decision making is based on these errors.

Behavioral economists have proposed a new approach that operates by "nudging" (Thaler & Sunstein, 2008) individual behavior toward self-interest. The approach attempts to influence people's choices in directions that will improve their lives via *choice architecture*. Choice architecture is a means of organizing choices in such a way that encourages people to make the healthiest decisions. The idea is based on the assumption that the environment influences the content of our choices. The approach has also been termed *libertarian paternalism*. It is intended to promote self-interested behavior without diminishing individuals' freedom to choose and to help those with self-control problems without distorting the decisions of those without such problems. The principles can be applied in both private and public sectors. For example, research has shown that by simply rearranging food items within a school (e.g., placing fruit at eye level, moving soda machines into more distant, inconvenient areas, or requiring students to pay cash for desserts and soft drinks) encourages children to buy more nutritious items (Wansink, 2006).[1] This strategy is much more effective than requiring students to eat vegetables. Moreover, when people feel as if they are freely and consciously making a choice, they take ownership of that decision and are more satisfied with the outcome.

THE PROBLEM OF TOO MUCH CHOICE

People with self-control problems may not behave in their own best interests. The purpose of self-control is to stabilize the choice in order to maximize long-term rewards. Common sense suggests that it is always preferred to have more options than fewer and better to have more knowledge than less. The rational model embraces the principle that expanding or improving the set of available alternatives necessarily makes an individual better off. However, people often seek means of restricting their own dietary choice. Thus, individuals may benefit from being constrained in their options.

We have an irrational compulsion to keep our options open, for example, when it comes to choosing a college major or involving our children in every activity we can imagine just in case one sparks interest. In these cases we ignore the consequences of indecision. We are spreading ourselves too thin. In fact we gain more by picking any option and sticking with it. More choice options are not always better. The philosopher Erich Fromm (1941) in his book *Escape from Freedom* writes that in modern society people are beset not by a lack of opportunity but by a dizzying abundance of it. What we need is to consciously start closing some of our options. Drop our commitments that are a waste of our time and use the energy on the option that should be left open. Barry Schwartz (2005) writes that the "excess of freedom" in today's Western cultures contributes to decreasing life satisfaction, increased depression, and sometimes paralysis.[2]

Increased consumer choices have been a mixed blessing. People who get to choose among 30 brands of jam or chocolate express less satisfaction than those who were only offered a half-dozen options (Schwartz, 2004). This "tyranny of choice" brings information overload and a greater likelihood that will feel regret over some of the unchosen options.

---

[1]For more information, see SmarterLunchrooms.org: http://www.smarterlunchrooms.org/research.html
[2]Starbucks Coffee Company brags that it presents customers with 19,000 options in each store.

In the book *The Challenge of Affluence,* Avner Offer (2007) argues that economic prosperity weakens self-control and undermines human well-being. The main reason is that choice is fallible. In particular, human beings want their pleasure now rather than tomorrow. The world is full of hyperbolic discounting. Obesity demonstrates how affluence reduces happiness. For example, Oswald and Powdthavee (2007) show that happiness is lower among heavier people. Stutzer (2007) shows that obesity is associated with reduced well-being, especially among a sub-sample of people who report that they have limited self-control.[3]

Engaging in good self-control can do more than protect people from bad outcomes. Human happiness is inseparable from self-control. The new and burgeoning field of positive psychology has recognized self-control as a vital human strength (Vohs et al., 2006). By forming our behavior into harmonious patterns through developing good habits we are able to maximize long-term rewards. Philosophers and religious leaders have been touting it since ancient times (Rachlin, 2000). Children better able to delay gratification were found to have better self-control and greater ability to regulate reactions to stress and frustration. Highly productive persons have better systems for self-control. So they waste less time on irrelevant goals. They often persist where others would quit. They develop the knack for enjoying unpleasantness. Thus, the purpose of self-control is not to deny ultimate pleasure but to increase it, regardless of the form that it takes.

Therefore policies that augment individuals' willpower would improve their well-being. For example, studies from the U.S. and Canada conclude that those with propensity to smoke are significantly happier with excise taxes rise (Gruber & Mullainathan, 2005). The results show that price increases can serve as a self-commitment device. Thus, tobacco taxes may not only serve as a means to generate revenue but may also help to overcome problems of self-control and prevent adolescents from starting a bad habit. That their satisfaction actually increased suggests that smoking was a choice they regretted and that they welcomed higher taxes as an aid to self-control.

CONCLUSION

This book presents a review of eating and obesity that are influenced by factors such as self-control problems, cognitive biases, and emotional influences. Hopefully, it has illustrated how the framework of behavioral

---

[3]However, this negative correlation between happiness and BMI does not establish causality. It is simply possible that unhappy people feel compelled to eat.

economics can be used to help consumers improve their dieting behavior and to enhance their well-being. The chapters focused on ways in which decision making can be impaired and strategies to improve decision making and willpower. The discussion dealt with the ability to pursue goals over long time spans, and the many ways in which the experience and the exertion of willful behavior can be disturbed. The understanding ways in which the decisions can be impaired or break down is a useful way to gain a better understanding of the nature of individual behavior. Rational persons may spend resources in an attempt to overcome their shortcomings. This means that rationality is not costless, but requires effort. The policy implication of this method is to help consumers help themselves by making more reasoned decisions.

References

Ainslie, G. (2001). *Breakdown of will*. Cambridge, NY: Cambridge University Press.

Akerlof, G. A., & Shiller, R. J. (2009). *Animal spirits: How human psychology drives the economy, and why it matters for global capitalism*. Princeton, NJ: Princeton University Press.

Almond, D. (2006). Is the 1918 influenza pandemic over? Long-term effects of in utero influenza exposure in the post-1940 U.S. population. *Journal of Political Economy, 114*, 672–712.

Alonso-Alonso, M., & Pascual-Leone, A. (2007). The right brain hypothesis for obesity. *Journal of the American Medical Association, 297*(16), 1819–1822.

American Psychiatric Association. (1993). Practice guideline for eating disorders. *American Journal of Psychiatry, 150*, 212–228.

American Psychiatric Association. (2000). *Diagnostic and statistical manual of mental disorders* (4th ed., Rev. text). Washington, DC: Author.

American Psychiatric Association Work Group on Eating Disorders. (2000). Practice guideline for the treatment of patients with eating disorders (revision). *American Journal of Psychiatry, 157*(Suppl. 1), 1–39.

Anderson, P. M., & Butcher, K. F. (2004). *Reading, writing and Raisinets: Are school finances contributing to children's obesity?* (WP 2004-16). Chicago, IL: Federal Reserve Bank of Chicago.

Andreyeva, T., Long, M. W., & Brownell, K. D. (2010). The impact of food prices on consumption: A systematic review of research on the price elasticity of demand for food. *American Journal of Public Health, 100*(2), 216–222.

Ariely, D. (2008). *Predictably irrational*. New York, NY: Harper Collins Publishers.

Arkes, J. (2001). *Does schooling improve adult health?* (Working Paper). Santa Monica, CA: RAND Corporation.

Atkins, R. C. (2002). *Dr. Atkins' new diet revolution* (2002 ed.). North Yorkshire, UK: Guill. 27.

Avena, N. M., Rada, P., & Hoebel, B. G. (2008). Evidence for sugar addiction: Behavioral and neurochemical effects of intermittent, excessive sugar intake. *Neuroscience and Biobehavioral Reviews, 32*, 20–39.

Ayers, I. (2010). *Carrots and sticks: Unlock the power of incentives to get things done*. New York, NY: Random House.

Bagwell, K. (2005). *The economic analysis of advertising* (Discussion Papers 0506-01). Columbia University, Department of Economics.

Bandura, A. (1997). *Self-efficacy: The exercise of control*. New York, NY: W. H. Freeman.

Bardone-Cone, A. M., Abramson, L. Y., Vohs, K. D., Heatherton, T. F., & Joiner, T. E. (2006). Predicting bulimic symptoms: An interactive model of self-efficacy, perfectionism, and perceived weight status. *Behaviour Research Therapy, 44*, 27–42.

Bargh, J. A., & Chartrand, T. L. (1999). The unbearable automaticity of being. *American Psychologist, 54,* 462–479.

Barker, D. J., Eriksson, J. G., Forsen, T., & Osmond, C. (2002). Fetal origins of adult disease: Strength of effects and biological basis. *International Journal for Epidemiology, 31*(6), 1235–1239.

Barnett, J. H., Salmond, C. H., Jones, P. B., & Sahakian, B. J. (2006). Cognitive reserve in neuropsychiatry. *Psychological Medicine, 36,* 1053–1064.

Barr-Anderson, D. J., Larson, N. I., Nelson, M. C., Neumark-Sztainer, D., & Story, M. (2009). Does television viewing predict dietary intake five years later in high school students and young adults? *International Journal of Behavioral Nutrition and Physical Activity, 6, 7.*

Baumeister, R. F. (2002). Yielding to temptation: Self-control failure, impulsive purchasing, and consumer behavior. *Journal of Consumer Research, 28,* 670–676.

Baumeister, R. F. (2005). *The cultural animal: Human nature, meaning, and social life.* New York, NY: Oxford University Press.

Baumeister, R. F., Dewall, C. N., Ciarocco, N. J., & Twenge, J. M. (2005). Social exclusion impairs self-regulation. *Journal of Personality and Social Psychology, 88,* 589–604.

Baumeister, R. F., Heatherton, T. F., & Tice, D. (1994). *Losing control: How and why people fail at self-regulation.* San Diego, CA: Academic Press.

Baumeister, R. F., Muraven, M., & Tice, D. M. (2000). Ego depletion: A resource model of volition, self-regulation and controlled processing. *Social Cognition, 18,* 130–150.

Baumeister, R. F., Sparks, E. A., Stillman, T. F., & Vohs, K. D. (2008). Free will in consumer behavior: Self-control, ego depletion and choice. *Journal of Consumer Psychology, 18,* 4 13.

Baumeister, R. F., Zell, A. L., & Tice, D. M. (2007). How emotions facilitate and impair self-regulation. In J. J. Gross (Ed.), *Handbook of emotion regulation* (pp. 408–426). New York, NY: Guilford Press.

Bechara, A. (2005). Decision making, impulse control and loss of willpower to resist drugs: Neurocognitive perspective. *Nature Neuroscience, 8*(11), 1458–1463.

Bechara, A., & Damasio, A. R. (2005). The somatic marker hypothesis: A neural theory of economic decision. *Games and Economic Behavior, 52,* 336–372.

Bechara, A., & Damasio, H. (2002). Decision-making and addiction (part I): Impaired activation of somatic states in substance dependent individuals when pondering decisions with negative future consequences. *Neuropsychologia, 40,* 1675–1689.

Becker, G. S. (1992). Habits, addictions and traditions. *Kyklos, 45*(3), 327–346.

Becker, G. S., & Mulligan, C. (1997). The endogenous determination of time preference. *Quarterly Journal of Economics, 112*(3), 729–758.

Benabou, R., & Tirole, J. (2002). Self-confidence and personal motivation. *Quarterly Journal of Economics, 117,* 871–915.

Benton, D. (2010). The plausibility of sugar addiction and its role in obesity and eating disorders. *Clinical Nutrition, 29,* 288–303.

Bernheim, B. D., & Rangel, A. (2004). Addiction and cue-conditioned cognitive processes. *American Economic Review, 94*(5), 1558–1590.

Berridge, K. C. (2004). Motivation concepts in behavioral neuroscience. *Physiology & Behavior, 81*(2), 179–209.

Berridge, K. C. (2007). The debate over dopamine's role in reward: The case for incentive salience. *Psychopharmacology, 191*(3), 391–431.

Berridge, K. C. (2009). 'Liking' and 'wanting' food rewards: Brain substrates and roles in eating disorders. *Physiology & Behavior, 97*(5), 537–550.

Berridge, K. C., Ho, C. Y., Richard, J. M., & DiFeliceantonio, A. G. (2010). The tempted brain eats: Pleasure and desire circuits in obesity and eating disorders. *Brain Research, 1350,* 43–64.

Beydoun M. A., Wang Y (2010). Pathways linking depression to SES, lifestyle factors and obesity among US adults. *Journal of Affective Disorders 123*(1–3):52–63.

Bhattacharya, J., & Sood, N. (2006). Health insurance and the obesity externality. *Advances in Health Economics and Health Services Research, The Economics of Obesity, 17,* 281–321.

Bickel, W. K., & Johnson, M. W. (2003). Junk time: Pathological behavior as the interaction of evolutionary and cultural forces. In N. Heather & R. Vuchinich (Eds.), *Choice, behavorial economics and addictions* (pp. 249–271). Amsterdam, The Netherlands: Pergamon.

Bickel, W. K., Miller, M. L., Yi, R., Kowal, B. P., Lindquist, D. M., & Pitcock, J. A. (2007). Behavioral and neuroeconomics of drug addiction: Competing neural systems and temporal discounting processes. *Drug and Alcohol Dependence, 90,* S85–S91.

Bickel, W. K., & Vuchinich, R. E. (2000). *Reframing health behavior change with behavioral economics.* Hillsdale, NJ: Lawrence Erlbaum Associates.

Blanchflower, D. G., Oswald, A. J., & van Landeghem, B. (2009). *Imitative obesity and relative utility* (IZA Discussion Paper Series No. 4010). Bonn, Germany: Institute for the Study of Labor.

Bleich, S., Cutler, D., Murray, C., & Adams, A. (2008). Why is the developed world obese? *Annual Review of Public Health, 29,* 273–295.

Boon, B., Stroebe, W., Schut, H., & Ijntema, R. (2002). Ironic processes in the eating behaviour of restrained eaters. *British Journal of Health Psychology, 7,* 1–10.

Bowers, D. E. (2000). Cooking trends echo changing roles of women. *FoodReview, 23*(1), 23–29.

Bray, G. A. (1998). Obesity: A time bomb to be defused. *Lancet, 352*(9123), 160–161.

Berridge, K. C. 'Liking' and 'wanting' food rewards: brain substrates and roles in eating disorders. *Physiology & Behavior, 97*(5), 537–550, 2009

Brown, A. J., Spanos, A., & Devlin, M. J. (2007). *Bulimia nervosa as an addiction: Evidence for a tolerance effect in patterns of binge eating over the course of illness.* Poster presented at the International Conference of Eating Disorders, Baltimore, MD.

Brownell, K. D., & Horgen, K. B. (2003). *Food fight: The inside story of the food industry, America's obesity crisis, and what we can do about it.* Chicago, IL: Contemporary Books.

Cacioppo, J. T., & Patrick, W. (2008). *Loneliness: Human nature and the need for social connection.* New York, NY: W. W. Norton.

Camerer, C., Loewenstein, G., & Rabin, M. (2003). *Advances in behavioral economics.* Princeton, NY: Princeton University Press.

Carrillo, J., & Mariotti, T. (2000). Strategic ignorance as a self-disciplining device. *Review of Economic Studies, 67,* 529–544.

Case, A., & Deaton, A. (2005). Broken down by work and sex: How our health declines. In D. A. Wise (Ed.), *Analyses in the economics of aging* (pp. 185–212). Chicago, IL: The University of Chicago Press.

Cassin, S. E., & von Ranson, K. M. (2007). Is binge eating experienced as an addiction? *Appetite, 49,* 687–690.

Caton, S. J., Ball, M., Ahern, A., & Hetherington, M. M. (2004). Dose-dependent effects of alcohol on appetite and food intake. *Physiology & Behavior, 81*(1), 51–58.

Cawley, J. (2004). The impact of obesity on wages. *Journal of Human Resources, 39,* 451–474.

Centers for Disease Control and Prevention. (2009). Cigarette smoking among adults and trends in smoking cessation—United States, 2008. *Morbidity and Mortality Weekly Report, 58,* 1227–1232.

Chaloupka, F. J., & Warner, K. E. (2000). The economics of smoking. In A. J. Culyer & J. P. Newhouse (Eds.), *Handbook of health economics* (Vol. 1, pp. 1539–1628). New York, NY: Elsevier.

Chen, Z., & Meltzer, D. (2008). Beefing up with the Chans: Evidence for the effects of relative income and income inequality on health from the China Health and Nutrition Survey. *Social Science & Medicine, 66,* 2206–2217.

Chou, S. Y., Grossman, M., & Saffer, H. (2004). An economic analysis of adult obesity: Results from the Behavioral Risk Factor Surveillance System. *Journal of Health Economics, 23*(3), 565–587.

Chou, S. Y., Rashad, I., & Grossman, M. (2008). Fast-food restaurant advertising on television and its influence on childhood obesity. *Journal of Law and Economics, 51,* 599–618.

Christakis, N. A., & Fowler, J. H. (2007). The spread of obesity in a large social network over 32 years. *New England Journal of Medicine, 357*(4), 370–379.

Christakis, N. A., & Fowler, J. H. (2009). *Connected: The surprising power of our social networks and how they shape our lives.* New York, NY: Little, Brown and Company.

Christian, T., & Rashad, I. (2009). Trends in U.S. food prices, 1950–2007 (with Thomas Christian). *Economics and Human Biology, 7*(1), 113–120.

Clauson, A., & Leibtag, E. (2008). *Food CPI, prices, and expenditures briefing room, table 12.* Washington, DC: U.S. Department of Agriculture, Economic Research Service.

Cocores, J. A., & Gold, M. S. (2009). The salted food addiction hypothesis may explain overeating and the obesity epidemic. *Medical Hypotheses, 73*(6), 892–899.

Coon, G. M., Pena, D., & Illich, P. A. (1998). Self-efficacy and substance abuse: Assessment using a brief phone interview. *Journal of Substance Abuse Treatment, 15,* 385–391.

Corwin, R. L., & Grigson, P. S. (2009). Symposium overview—Food addiction: Fact or fiction? *The Journal of Nutrition, 139,* 617–619.

Courtemanche, C. (2009). Longer hours and larger waistlines? The relationship between work hours and obesity. *Forum for Health Economics & Policy, 12*(2), pp. 1–31.

Crockett, M. J., Clark, L., Tabibnia, G., Lieberman, M. D., & Robbins, T. W. (2008). Serotonin modulates behavioral reactions to unfairness. *Science, 320*(5884), 1739.

Currie, J., & Moretti, E. (2003). Mother's education and the intergenerational transmission of human capital: Evidence from college openings. *Quarterly Journal of Economics, 118*(4), 1495–1532.

Currie, J., Vigna, S. D., Moretti, E., & Pathania, V. (2009). *The effect of fast food restaurants on obesity* (Working Paper No. 14721). Cambridge, MA: National Bureau of Economic Research.

Cutler, D., Glasser, E. L., & Shapiro, J. M. (2003). Why have Americans become more obese? *The Journal of Economic Perspectives, 17*(3), 93–118.

Cutler, D. M., Lleras-Muney, A., & Vogl, T. (2010). *Socioeconomic status and health: Dimensions and mechanisms.* New York, NY: Oxford Handbook of Health Economics.

Dabelea, D., Hanson, R. L., Bennett, P. H., Roumain, J., Knowler, W. C., & Pettitt, D. J. (1998). Increasing prevalence of Type II diabetes in American Indian children. *Diabetologia, 41,* 904–910.

Dagher, A. (2009). The neurobiology of appetite: Hunger as addiction. *International Journal of Obesity (London), 33*(Suppl. 2), S30–S33.

Dallman, M. F. (2010). Stress-induced obesity and the emotional nervous system. *Trends in Endocrinology & Metabolism, 21,* 159–165.

Dallman, M. F., Pecoraro, N. C., & la Fleur, S. E. (2005). Chronic stress and comfort foods: Self-medication and abdominal obesity. *Brain, Behavior, and Immunity, 19,* 275–280.

Damasio, A. R. (1994). *Descartes' error: Emotion, reason, and the human brain.* New York, NY: G. P. Putnam.

Damasio, A. R. (1999). *The feeling of what happens: Body and emotion in the making of consciousness.* San Diego, CA: Harcourt.

Darmon, N., & Drewnowski, A. (2008). Does social class predict diet quality? *American Journal of Clinical Nutrition, 88*(4), 1177–1178.

Datar, A., & Sturm, R. (2006). Childhood overweight and elementary school outcomes. *International Journal of Obesity, 30,* 1449–1460.

Davidson, R. J., & Irwin, W. (1999). The functional neuroanatomy of emotion and affective style. *Trends in Cognitive Sciences, 3,* 11–21.

Davis, C., Patte, K., Levitan, R., Reid, C., Tweed, S., & Curtis, C. (2007). From motivation to behaviour: Model of reward sensitivity, overeating, and food preferences in the risk profile for obesity. *Appetite, 48*(1), 12–19.

Davis, C., Strachan, S., & Berkson, M. (2004). Sensitivity to reward: Implications for overeating and overweight. *Appetite, 42,* 131–138.

Deaton, Angus (2003). Health, inequality and economic development. *Journal of Economic Literature, 41*(1), 113–158.

Deci, E. L., & Ryan, R. M. (2000). The "what" and "why" of goal pursuits: Human needs and the self-determination of behavior. *Psychological Inquiry, 11,* 227–268.

DellaVigna, S., & Malmendier, U. (2006, forthcoming). Paying not to go to the gym. *American Economic Review, 90*(3), 694–719.

DelParigi, A., Chen, K., Salbe, A. D., Hill, J. O., Wing, R. R., Reiman, E. M., & Tataranni, P. (2007). Successful dieters have increased neural activity in cortical areas involved in the control of behavior. *International Journal of Obesity (London), 31*(3), 440–448.

DeWall, C. N. (2009). Rejection. In H. T. Reis & S. Sprecher (Eds.), *Encyclopedia of human relationships.* Thousand Oaks, CA: Sage.

DHHS (U.S. Department of Health and Human Services). (2000). *Healthy people 2010: Understanding and improving health* (2nd ed.). Washington, DC: U.S.

Government Printing Office. Retrieved October 13, 2010, from http://www.healthypeople.gov/publications

Dingemans, A., Martijn, C., Jansen, A. T. M., & van Furth, E. F. (2009). The effect of suppressing negative emotions on eating behavior in binge eating disorder. *Appetite, 52*(1), 51–57.

Doblhammer, G. (2004). *The late life legacy of very early life* (Demographic Research Monographs). New York, NY: Springer.

Downs, J. S., Loewenstein, G., & Wisdom, J. (2009a). Eating by the numbers. *New York Times*, p. A31.

Downs, J. S., Loewenstein, G., & Wisdom, J. (2009b). Strategies for promoting healthier food choices. *American Economic Review, 99*(2), 159–164.

Drewnowski, A. (1997). Taste preferences and food intake. *Annual Review of Nutrition, 17*, 237–253.

Drewnowski, A., & Darmon, N. (2005). Food choices and diet costs: An economic analysis. *Journal of Nutrition, 135*(4), 900–904.

Dunham, D. (1994). *Food costs from farm to retail in 1993*. Washington, DC: USDA Economic Research Service.

Elfhag, K., & Rossner, S. (2005). Who succeeds in maintaining weight loss? A conceptual review of factors associated with weight loss maintenance and weight regain. *Obesity Review, 6*(1), 67–85.

Ellis, A. (2005). Discussion of Christine A. Padesky and Aaron T. Beck, "Science and philosophy: Comparison of cognitive therapy and rational emotive behavior therapy." *Journal of Cognitive Psychotherapy, 19*(2), 181–185.

Elster, J. (1989). Social norms and economic theory. *Journal of Economic Perspectives, 3*, 99–117.

Elster, J. (1999a). *Alchemies of the mind*. New York, NY: Oxford University Press.

Elster, J. (1999b). *Strong feelings: Emotion, addiction, and human behavior*. Cambridge, MA: The MIT Press.

Elster, J. (2001). Introduction. In J. Elster (Ed.), *Addiction: Entries and exits*. New York, NY: Russell Sage Foundation.

Elster, J. (2006). Weakness of will and preference reversal. In J. Elster, O. Gjelsvik, A. Hylland, & K. Moene (Eds.), *Understanding choice, explaining behavior: Essays in honour of Ole-Jørgen Skog*. Oslo, Norway: Oslo Academic Press.

Elster, J., & Skog, O. J. (2000). *Getting hooked: Rationality and addiction*. Cambridge, UK: Cambridge University Press.

Epstein, S. (1994). Integration of the cognitive and psychodynamic unconscious. *American Psychologist, 49*, 709–724.

Epstein, L. H., Roemmich, J. N., Robinson, J. L., Paluch, R. A., Winiewicz, D. D., Fuerch, J. H., & Robinson, T. N. (2008). A randomized trial of the effects of reducing television viewing and computer use on body mass index in young children. *Archives of Pediatrics Adolescent Medicine, 162*(3), 239–245.

Epstein, L. H., Temple, J. L., Roemmich, J. N., & Bouton, M. E. (2009). Habituation as a determinant of human food intake. *Psychological Review, 116*, 384–407.

Evans, J. St. B. T. (2008). Dual-processing accounts of reasoning, judgment, and social cognition. *Annual Review of Psychology, 59*, 6.1–6.24.

Ezzati, M., Lopez, A. D., Rodgers, A., Hoorn, S., & Murray, C. J. (2002). Selected major risk factors and global and regional burden of disease. *Lancet, 360*, 1347–1360.

Fedoroff, I., Polivy, J., & Herman, C. P. (1997). The effect of pre-exposure to food cues on the eating behavior of restrained and unrestrained eaters. *Appetite, 28,* 33–47.

Feldstein, P. J. (2007). *Health policy issues: An economic perspective* (4th ed.). Chicago, IL: Health Administration Press.

Field, M., & Cox, W. M. (2008). Attentional bias in addictive behaviors: A review of its development, causes, and consequences. *Drug and Alcohol Dependence, 97,* 1–20.

Field, A. E., Javaras, K. M., Aneja, P., Kitos, N., Camargo, C. A., Taylor, C. B., & Laird, N. M. (2008). Family, peer, and media predictors of becoming eating disordered. *Archives of Pediatrics & Adolescent Medicine, 162*(6), 574–579.

Finlayson, G., King, N., & Blundell, J. E. (2007). Is it possible to dissociate 'liking' and 'wanting' for foods in humans? A novel experimental procedure. *Physiology & Behavior, 90,* 36–42.

Finkelstein, E. A., Ruhm, C. J., & Kosa, K. M. (2005). Economic causes and consequences of obesity. *Annual Review of Public Health, 26,* 239–257.

Finkelstein, E. A., Trogdon, J. G., Cohen, J. W., & Dietz, W. (2009). Annual medical spending attributable to obesity: Payer- and service-specific estimates. *Health Affairs, 28,* w822–w831.

Finucane, M. L., Alhakami, A., Slovic, P., & Johnson, S. M. (2000). The affect heuristic in judgments of risk and benefits. *Journal of Behavioral Decision Making, 13,* 1–17.

Fishbach, A., Friedman, R. S., & Kruglanski, A. W. (2003). Leading us not into temptation: Momentary allurements elicit overriding goals activation. *Journal of Personality and Social Psychology, 84,* 296–309.

Fishbach, A., & Shah, J. Y. (2006). Self-control in action: Implicit dispositions toward goals and away from temptations. *Journal of Personality and Social Psychology, 90,* 820–832.

Flegal, K. M., Carroll, M. D., Ogden, C. L., & Curtin, L. R. (2010). Prevalence and trends in obesity among US adults, 1999–2008. *Journal of the American Medical Association, 303*(3), 235–241.

Flegal, K. M., & Troiano, R. P. (2000). Changes in the distribution of body mass index of adults and children in the US population. *International Journal of Obesity and Related Metabolic Disorders, 24,* 807–818.

Fox, J. A., Hayes, D. J., & Shogren, J. F. (2002). Consumer preferences for food irradiation. *The Journal of Risk and Uncertainty, 24,* 75–95.

Frank, R. H. (2003). *Microeconomics and behavior.* New York, NY: McGraw-Hill.

French, S. A., Jeffery, R. W., Story, M., Breitlow, K. K., Baxter, J. S., Hannan, P., & Snyder, M. P. (2001). Pricing and promotion effects on low-fat vending snack purchases: The CHIPS study. *American Journal of Public Health, 91,* 112–117.

Freud, S. (1924/1962). *The ego and the id* (J. Riviere, Trans.). New York, NY: W. W. Norton.

Fromm, E. (1941). *Escape from freedom.* New York, NY: Holt, Rinehart, and Winston.

Fuchs, V. R. (1986). Economics, health, and postindustrial society. In V. R. Fuchs (Eds.), *The health economy* (pp. 153–182). Cambridge, MA: Harvard University Press. Originally published in the *Milbank Memorial Fund Quarterly/Health and Society, 57* (Spring 1979).

Gailliot, M. T., & Baumeister, R. F. (2007). The physiology of willpower: Linking blood glucose to Self-control. *Personality and Social Psychology Review, 11,* 303–327.

Gailliot, M. T., Plant, E. A., Butz, D. A., & Baumeister, R. F. (2007). Self-control relies on glucose as a limited energy source: Willpower is more than a metaphor. *Journal of Personality and Social Psychology, 92,* 325–336.

Gallagher, M. (2006). *Research and consulting group.* Retrieved from http://www.agr.state.il.us/marketing/ILOFFTaskForce/ChicagoFoodDesertReportFull.pdf

Gallo, L. C., Bogart, L. M., Vranceanu, A. M., & Matthews, K. A. (2005). Socioeconomic status, resources, psychological experiences, and emotional responses: A test of the reserve capacity model. *Journal of Personality and Social Psychology, 88*(2), 386–399.

Garrow, J. S. (1988). *Obesity and related diseases.* Edinburgh, UK: Churchill Livingstone.

Gaviria, A., & Raphael, S. (2001). School-based peer effects and juvenile behavior. *Review of Economics and Statistics, 83*(2), 257–268.

Gazzaniga, M. S. (2005). *The ethical brain.* New York, NY: DANA Press.

Gazzaniga, M. S. (2008). *Human: The science behind what makes us unique.* New York, NY: HarperCollins.

Gearhardt, A. N., Corbin, W. R., & Brownell, K. D. (2009). Preliminary validation of the Yale food addiction scale. *Appetite, 52*(2), 430–436.

Geier, A. B., Foster, G. D., Womble, L. G., McLaughlin, J., Borradaile, K. E., Nachmani, J., . . . Shults, J. (2007). The relationship between relative weight and school attendance among elementary schoolchildren. *Obesity, 15*(8), 2157–2161.

Gladwell, M. (2005). *Blink: The power of thinking without thinking.* New York, NY: Little, Brown & Company.

Gladwell, M. (2008). *Outliers: The story of success.* New York, NY: Little, Brown & Company.

Goldbeck, R., Myatt, P., & Aitchison, T. (1997). End-of-treatment self-efficacy: A predictor of abstinence. *Addiction, 92,* 313–324.

Goldberg, E. (2009). *The new executive brain: Frontal lobes in a complex world.* New York, NY: Oxford University Press.

Goldman, D. P., Lakdawalla, D. N., & Zheng, Y. (2009). Food prices and the dynamics of body weight. In M. Grossman & N. Mocan (Eds.), *Economic aspects of obesity.* Chicago, IL: University of Chicago Press.

Gollwitzer, P. M. (1993). Goal achievement: The role of intentions. *European Review of Social Psychology, 4,* 141–185.

Gollwitzer, P. M., Gawrilow, C., & Oettingen, G. (2010). The power of planning: Self-control by effective goal-striving. In R. R. Hassin, K. N. Ochsner, & Y. Trope (Eds.), *Self control in society, mind, and brain* (pp. 279–296). New York, NY: Oxford University Press.

Gollwitzer, P. M., & Sheeran, P. (2006). Implementation intentions and goal achievement: A meta-analysis of effects and processes. *Advances in Experimental Social Psychology, 38,* 69–119.

Gortmaker, S. L., Must, A., Perrin, J. A., Sobol, A. M., & Dietz, W. H. (1993). Social and economic consequences of overweight in adolescence and young adulthood. *New England Journal of Medicine, 329,* 1008–1012.

Green, L., Fry, A. F., & Myerson, J. (1994). Discounting of delayed rewards: A life-span comparison. *Psychological Science, 5*, 33–36.

Grossman, M. (1972). On the concept of health capital and the demand for health. *Journal of Political Economy, 80*(2), 223–249.

Gruber, J. H., & Mullainathan, S. (2005). Do cigarette taxes make smokers happier? *Advances in Economic Analysis and Policy, 5*(1), 1–43.

Guerrieri, R., Nederkoorn, C., Stankiewicz, K., Alberts, H., Geschwind, N., Martijn, C., & Jansen, A. (2007). The influence of trait and induced state impulsivity on food intake in normal-weight healthy women. *Appetite, 49*, 66–73.

Gunstad, J., Paul, R. H., Cohen, R. A., Tate, D. F., Spitznagel, M. B., & Gordon, E. (2007). Elevated body mass index is associated with executive dysfunction in otherwise healthy adults. *Comprehensive Psychiatry, 48*(1), 57–61.

Guthrie, J. F., Lin, B. H., & Frazao, E. (2002). Role of food prepared away from home in the American diet, 1977–78 versus 1994–96: Changes and consequences. *Journal of Nutrition Education and Behavior, 34*(3), 140–150.

Hammond, R. A. (2009). Complex systems modeling for obesity research. *Preventing Chronic Disease, 6*(3). Retrieved from http://www.cdc.gov/pcd/issues/2009/jul/09_0017.htm

Harris, J. L., Brownell, K. D., & Bargh, J. A. (2009). The food marketing defense model: Integrating psychological research to protect youth and inform public policy. *Social Issues and Policy Review, 3*(1), 211–271.

Harrison, D. M. (2008). Oral sucrose for pain management for infants: Myths and misconceptions. *Journal of Neonatal Nursing, 14*, 39–46.

Healthy People 2010 (2nd ed.). (2000). Washington, DC: U.S. Government Printing Office.

Hebb, D. O. (1949). *The organization of behavior.* New York, NY: Wiley.

Hebl, M. R., & Mannix, L. M. (2003). The weight of obesity in evaluating others: A mere proximity effect. *Personality and Social Psychology Bulletin, 29*, 28–38.

Heckman, J. J. (2007). The economics, technology, and neuroscience of human capacity formation. *Proceedings of the National Academy of Sciences of the United States of America, 104*(33), 13240–13255.

Herman, C. P., & Polivy, J. (1980). Restrained eating. In A. J. Stunkard (Ed.), *Obesity* (pp. 208–225). Philadelphia, PA: W. B. Saunders.

Herman, C. P., & Polivy, J. (1984). A boundary model for the regulation of eating. In A. J. Stunkard & E. Stellar (Eds.), *Eating and its disorders* (pp. 141–156). New York, NY: Raven Press.

Herman, C. P., & Polivy, J. (2002). Dieting as exercise in behavioral economics. In G. Loewenstein, R. Baumeister, & D. Read (Eds.), *Time and decision*. New York, NY: Russell Sage Foundation.

Herman, C. P., & Polivy, J. (2008). External cues in the control of food intake in humans: The sensory-normative distinction. *Physiology & Behavior, 94*, 722–728.

Herman, C. P., Roth, D. A., & Polivy, J. (2003). Social influences on eating: A review of the literature. *Psychological Bulletin, 129*, 873–886.

Heshka, S., Anderson, J. W., Atkinson, R. L., Greenway, F. L., Hill, J. O., Phinney, S. D., . . . Pi-Sunyer, F. X. (2003). Weight loss with self-help compared with a structured commercial program: A randomized trial. *The Journal of the American Medical Association, 289*, 1792–1798.

Heyman, G. M. (2009). *Addiction: A disorder of choice.* Cambridge, MA: Harvard University Press.

Higgins, E. T. (1996). The "self digest": Self-knowledge serving self-regulatory functions. *Journal of Personality and Social Psychology, 71,* 1062–1083.

Hill, J., & Peters, J. (1998). Environmental contributions to the obesity epidemic. *Science, 280*(5368), 1371–1374.

Hoch, S. J., & Loewenstein, G. (1991, March). Time-inconsistent preferences and consumer self-control. *Journal of Consumer Research, 17,* 492–507.

Hoebel, B. G. (1999). Neural systems for reinforcement and inhibition of behavior: Relevance to eating, addiction and depression. In D. Kahneman, E. Diener, & N. Schwarz (Eds.), *Understanding quality of life: Scientific perspectives on enjoyment and suffering.* New York, NY: Russell Sage Foundation.

Hoebel, B. G., Rada, P. V., Mark, G. P., & Pothos, E. (1999). Neural systems for reinforcement and inhibition of behavior: Relevance to eating, addiction and depression. In D. Kahneman, E. Diener, & N. Schwarz (Eds.), *Well-being: Foundations of hedonic psychology* (pp. 560–574). New York: Russell Sage Foundation.

Hoebel, B. G., Avena, N. M., & Rada, P. (2007). Accumbens dopamine-acetylcholine balance in approach and avoidance. *Current Opinion in Pharmacology, 7,* 617–627.

Hoebel, B. G., Bartley, G., Avena, N. M., Bocarsly, M. E., & Rada, P. (2009). Natural addiction: A behavioral and circuit model based on sugar addiction in rats. *Journal of Addiction Medicine, 3,* 33–41.

Hogarth, R. M. (2001). *Educating intuition.* Chicago, IL: The University of Chicago Press.

Holton, R. (2003). How is strength of will possible? In S. Stroud & C. Tappolet (Eds.), *Weakness of will and practical irrationality* (pp. 39–67). Oxford, NY: Clarendon Press.

Holton, R. (2009). *Willing, wanting, waiting.* New York, NY: Oxford University Press.

Hu, F. B. (2008). *Obesity epidemiology.* New York, NY: Oxford University Press.

Hudson, J. I., & Pope, H. G. (2007). Genetic epidemiology of eating disorders and co-occurring conditions: The role of endophenotypes. *International Journal of Eating Disorders, 40*(Suppl.), S76–S78.

Iacoboni, M. (2008). *Mirroring people: The new science of how we connect with others.* New York, NY: Farrar, Straus & Giroux.

Ifland, J. R., Preuss, H. G., Marcus, M. T., Rourke, K. M., Taylor, W. C., Burau, K., . . . Manso, G. (2009). Refined food addiction: A classic substance use disorder. *Medical Hypotheses, 72*(5): 518–526.

Institute of Medicine. (2003). *Weight management: State of the science and opportunities for military programs.* Washington, DC: The National Academy Press.

Institute of Medicine. (2004). *Exploring a vision: Integrating knowledge for food and health.* Washington, DC: The National Academy of Sciences.

Institute of Medicine. (2006). National academy of sciences, committee on food marketing and the diets of children and youth. In J. M. McGinnis, J. Gootman, & V. I. Kraak (Eds.), *Food marketing to children and youth: Threat or opportunity?* Washington, DC: Institute of Medicine of the National Academies.

Jabs, J., & Devine, C. M. (2006). Time scarcity and food choices: An overview. *Appetite, 47*, 196–204.

James, M. (2003). *Memory and emotion: The making of lasting memories*. New York, NY: Columbia University Press.

Johnson, E. J., & Goldstein, D. (2003). Do defaults save lives? *Science, 302*, 1338–1339.

Just, D. R., Mancino, L., & Wansink, B. (2007). *Could behavioral economics help improve diet quality for nutrition assistance program participants?* (Economic Research Report no. 43). Washington, DC: U.S. Department of Agriculture, Economic Research Service.

Kabat-Zinn, J. (1994). *Wherever you go there you are: Mindfulness meditation in everyday life*. New York, NY: Hyperion.

Kahneman, D. (2000). Experienced utility and objective happiness: A moment-based approach. In D. Kahneman & A. Tversky (Eds.), *Choices, values and frames* (pp. 673–692). New York, NY: Cambridge University Press and the Russell Sage Foundation.

Kahneman, D. (2003). Maps of bounded rationality: Psychology for behavioral economics, *American Economic Review, American Economic Association, 93*(5), 1449–1475.

Kahneman, D., Schkade, D. A., Fischler, C., Krueger, A. B., & Krilla, A. (2009). The structure of well-being in two cities: Life satisfaction and experienced happiness in Columbus, Ohio; and Rennes, France. In E. Diener, J. F. Helliwell, & D. Kahneman (Eds.), *International differences in well-being*. New York, NY: Oxford University Press.

Kaye, W. (2008). Neurobiology of anorexia and bulimia nervosa. *Physiology & Behavior, 94*, 121–135.

Keel, P. D., Dorer, D., Franko, S., Jackson, S., & Herzog, D. (2005). Postremission predictors of replace in women with eating disorders. *American Journal of Psychiatry, 162*, 2263–2268.

Keenan, P. S. (2009). Effect of new diagnoses on smoking and weight change. *Archives of Internal Medicine, 169*, 237.

Kelley, A. E. (2004). Ventral striatal control of appetitive motivation: Role in ingestive behavior and reward-related learning. *Neuroscience & Biobehavioral Reviews, 27*, 765–776.

Kersh, R., & Morone, J. (2002). The politics of obesity: Seven steps to government action. *Health Affairs, 21*(6), 162–175.

Kessler, D. (2009). *The end of overeating: Taking control of the insatiable American Appetite*. Rodale Books.

Keys, A., Brozek, J., Henschel, A., Mickelsen, O., & Taylor, H. L. (1950). *The biology of human starvation*. Oxford, MN: University of Minnesota Press.

Kirby, K. N., & Guastello, B. (2001). Making choices in anticipation of similar future choices can increase self-control. *Journal of Experimental Psychology: Applied, 7*, 154–164.

Kivetz, R., & Zheng, Y. (2006). Determinants of justification and self-control. *Journal of Experimental Psychology: General, 135*(4), 572–587.

Klein, N. (1999). *No logo: Taking aim at the brand bullies*. New York, NY: Picador.

Kolata, G. (2007). *Rethinking thin: The new science of weight loss—and the myths and realities of dieting*. New York, NY: Farrar, Straus and Giroux.

Koob, G. F. (2003). Drug reward and addiction. In L. R. Squire, F. E. Bloom, & S. K. McConnell (Eds.), *Fundamental neuroscience* (2nd ed., p. 1127). San Diego, CA: Academic Press.

Koob, G. F., & Le Moal, M. (2005). *Neurobiology of addiction.* San Diego, CA: Academic Press.

Kronick, I., & Knauper, B. (2010). Temptations elicit compensatory intentions. *Appetite, 54*(2), 398–401.

Kuijer, R., de Ridder, D., Ouwehand, C., Houx, B., & van den Bos, R. (2008). Dieting as a case of behavioural decision making: Does self-control matter? *Appetite, 51,* 506–511.

Laibson, D. (1997). Golden eggs and hyperbolic discounting. *Quarterly Journal of Economics, 112,* 443–478.

Laibson, D. (2001). A cue-theory of consumption. *Quarterly Journal of Economics, 66*(1), 81–120.

LeDoux, J. E. (1996). *The emotional brain: The mysterious underpinnings of emotional life.* New York, NY: Simon & Schuster.

LeDoux, J. (2002). *Synaptic self.* New York, NY: Viking.

Lenton, A. P., & Francesconi, M. (2010). How humans cognitively manage an abundance of mate options. *Psychological Science, 21,* 528–533.

Leshner, A. (1997). Addiction is a brain disease and it matters. *Science, 278,* 45–47.

Li, Y., Dai, Q., Jackson, J. C., & Zhang, J. (2008). Overweight is associated with decreased cognitive functioning among school-age children and adolescents. *Obesity (Silver Spring), 16*(8), 1809–1815.

Liu, W., & Aaker, J. (2008). The happiness of giving: The think time-ask effect. *Journal of Consumer Research, 35,* 543–557.

Loewenstein, G. (1996). Out of control: Visceral influences on behavior. *Organizational Behavior and Human Decision Processes, 65,* 272–292.

Loewenstein, G. (1999). A visceral theory of addiction. In J. Elster & O. J. Skog (Eds.), *Getting hooked: Rationality and the addictions.* Cambridge, UK: Cambridge University Press.

Loewenstein, G., O'Donoghue, T., & Rabin, M. (2003). Projection bias in predicting future utility. *Quarterly Journal of Economics, 118*(4), 1209–1248.

Loewenstein, G., Read, D., & Baumeister, R. F. (Eds.). (2003). *Time and decision: Economic and psychological perspectives on intertemporal choice.* New York, NY: Russell Sage Foundation.

Loewenstein, G., Weber, E. U., & Hsee, C. K. (2001). Risk as feelings. *Psychological Bulletin, 127*(2), 267–286.

Logue, A. W. (1988). Research on self-control: An integrating framework. *Behavioral and Brain Sciences, 11,* 665–709.

Lowe, M. R. (2003). Self-regulation of energy intake in the prevention and treatment of obesity: Is it feasible? *Obesity Research, 11*(10), 44S–59S.

Lowe, M. R., & Butryn, M. L. (2007). Hedonic hunger: A new dimension of appetite? *Physiology & Behavior, 91*(4), 432–439.

Lowe, M. R., & Kral, T. V. E. (2006). Stress-induced eating in restrained eaters may not be caused by stress or restraint. *Appetite, 46,* 16–21.

Lowe, M. R., van Steenburgh, J., Ochner, C., & Coletta, M. (2009). Neural correlates of individual differences related to appetite. *Physiology & Behavior, 97,* 561–571.

Madden, G. J., & Bickel, W. K. (2010). *Impulsivity: The behavioral and neurological science of discounting.* Washington, DC: American Psychological Association.

Mancino, L., & Kinsey, J. (2004). *Diet quality and calories consumed: The impact of being hungrier, busier and eating out* (WP-04-02). St. Paul, MN: The Food Industry Center, University of Minnesota.

Mann, T., Tomiyama, J., Westling, E., Lew, A. M., Samuels, B., & Chatman, J. (2007). Medicare's search for effective obesity treatments: Diets are not the answer. *American Psychologist, 62,* 220–233.

Marcenko, M. O., Kemp, S. P., & Larson, N. C. (2000). Childhood experiences of abuse, later substance use, and parenting outcomes among low-income mothers. *American Journal of Orthopsychiatry, 70,* 316–326.

Marlatt, A. G., & Witkewitz, K. (2005). Relapse prevention for alcohol and drug problem. In G. A. Marlatt & D. M. Donovan (Eds.), *Maintenance strategies in the treatment of addictive behaviors.* New York, NY: The Guilford Press.

Marmot, M. G. (2006). Status syndrome: A challenge to medicine. *Journal of the American Medical Association, 295*(11), 1304–1307.

Marmot, M. G., & Bell, R. (2009). Action on health disparities in the United States: Commission on social determinants of health. *Journal of the American Medical Association, 301,* 1169–1171.

May, R. (1999). *Freedom and destiny.* New York, NY: W. W. Norton (Original work published 1981).

Mazzocchi, M., Traill, W. B., & Shogren, J. F. (2009). *Fat economics: Nutrition, health, and economic policy.* New York, NY: Oxford University Press.

McCabe, K. (2003). Neuroeconomics. In L. Nadel (Ed.), *The encyclopedia of cognitive science* (Vol. 3, pp. 294–298). New York, NY: Nature Publishing Group, Macmillan Publishers Ltd.

McCarty, C. A., Kosterman, R., Mason, W. A., & McCauley, E. (2009). Longitudinal associations among depression, obesity and alcohol use disorders in young adulthood. *General Hospital Psychiatry, 31*(5), 442–450.

McClure, S. M., Laibson, D. I., Loewenstein, G., & Cohen, J. D. (2004). Separate neural systems value immediate and delayed monetary rewards. *Science, 306*(15), 503–507.

McEwen, B. S. (1998). Protective and damaging effects of stress mediators. *New England Journal of Medicine, 338*(3), 171–179.

McGaugh, J. L. (2003). *Memory and emotion: The making of lasting memories.* New York, NY: Columbia University Press.

McGinnis, J. M. (1999). *Causes of morbidity and mortality in the United States: Report to the Robert Wood Johnson foundation.* Princeton, NJ: Robert Wood Johnson Foundation.

McGinnis, J. M., & Foege, W. H. (1993). Actual causes of death in the United States. *Journal of the American Medical Association, 270*(18), 207–212.

McGuire, M. T., Wing, R. R., Klem, M. L., Lang, W., & Hill, J. O. (1999). What predicts weight regain in a group of successful weight losers? *Journal of Consulting and Clinical Psychology, 67*(2), 177–185.

Mennella, J. A., Jagnow, C. J., & Beauchamp, G. K. (2001). Pre- and post-natal flavor learning by human infants. *Pediatrics, 107,* e88.

Metcalfe, J., & Mischel, W. (1999). A hot/cool-system analysis of delay of gratification: Dynamics of willpower. *Psychological Review, 106*(1), 3–19.

Miller, D. L., Page, M. E., Stevens, A. H., & Filipski, M. (2009). Why are recessions good for your health? *American Economic Review: Papers & Proceedings, 99*(2), 122–127.

Mischel, W., & Ayduk, O. (2004). Willpower in a cognitive–affective–processing system: The dynamics of delay of gratification. In R. F. Baumeister & K. D. Vohs (Eds.), *Handbook of self regulation: Research, theory, and applications* (pp. 99–129). New York, NY: Guilford Press.

Mischel, W., Shoda, Y., & Peake, P. K. (1988). The nature of adolescent competencies predicted by preschool delay of gratification. *Journal of Personality and Social Psychology, 54*, 687–696.

Mocan, N. H., & Tekin, E. (2009). *Obesity, self-esteem and wages* (Working Paper No. 15101). Cambridge, MA: National Bureau of Economic Research.

Muraven, M. (2008). Autonomous self-control is less depleting. *Journal of Research in Personality, 42*, 763–770.

Murphy, K. M., & Topel, R. H. (2005, Winter). Black-white differences in the economic value of improving health. *Perspectives Biology and Medicine, 48*(Suppl.), S176–S194.

National Association of State Mental Health Program Directors: Medical Directors Council. (2008). *Measurement of health status for people with serious mental illness.* Alexandria, VA: Author.

Naqvi, N. H., & Bechara, A. (2009). The hidden island of addiction: The insula. *Trends in Neurosciences, 32*(1), 56–67.

Naqvi, N. H., Rudrauf, D., Damasio, H., & Bechara, A. (2007). Damage to the insula disrupts addiction to cigarette smoking. *Science, 315*, 531–534.

National Eating Disorders Association (NEDA). (2008). Retrieved from http://www.nationaleatingdisorders.org/uploads/file/toolkits/NEDA-Toolkit-Educators_09-15-08.pdf

National Institute of Mental Health. (2006). *College women at risk for eating disorder may benefit from online intervention.* Retrieved from http://www.nimh.nih.gov/science-news/2006/college-women-at-risk-for-eating-disorder-may-benefit-from-online-intervention.shtml

National Youth Risk Behavior Survey. (2005). Retrieved from http://www.cdc.gov/HealthyYouth/yrbs/index.htm

Neel, J. V. (1962). Diabetes mellitus: A "thrifty" genotype rendered detrimental by "progress?" *American Journal of Human Genetics, 14*, 353–362.

Nestle, M. (2002). *Food politics: How the food industry influences nutrition and health.* Berkeley, CA: University of California Press.

Nestler, E. J., & Malenka, R. C. (2004, March). The addicted brain. *Scientific American, 290*(3), 78–85.

Nijs, I. M., Muris, P., Euser, A. S., & Franken, I. H. (2009). Differences in attention to food and food intake between overweight/obese and normal-weight females under conditions of hunger and satiety. *Appetite, 54*(2), 243–254.

Nord, M. (2009). *Food insecurity in households with children: Prevalence, severity, and household characteristics* (EIB-56). Washington, DC: USDA, Economic Research Service. Retrieved from www.ers.usda.gov/publications/eib56/

North, A. C., Hargreaves, D. J., & McKendrick, J. (1997). In-store music affects product choice. *Nature, 390,* 132.

O'Donoghue, T., & Rabin, M. (1999). Doing it now or later. *American Economic Review, 89,* 103–124.

Oettingen, G., & Gollwitzer, P. M. (2010). Strategies of setting and implementing goals: Mental contrasting and implementation intentions. In J. E. Maddux & J. P. Tangney (Eds.), *Social psychological foundations of clinical psychology* (pp. 114–135). New York, NY: Guilford Press.

Offer, A. (2006). *The challenge of affluence: Self-control and well-being in the United States and Britain since 1950.* New York, NY: Oxford University Press.

Okada, E. M. (2006). Justification effects on consumer choice of hedonic and utilitarian goods. *Journal of Marketing Research, 42*(1), 43–53.

Oliver, J. E., & Lee, T. (2005). Public opinion and the politics of obesity in America. *Journal of Health Politics, Policy, and Law, 30,* 923–954.

Oswald, A. J., & Powdthavee, N. (2007). Obesity, unhappiness, and the challengeof affluence: Theory and evidence. *Economic Journal, 117,* F441–F454.

Otsuka, R., Tamakoshi, K., Yatsuya, H., Murata, C., Sekiya, A., ada, K., . . . Toyoshima, H. (2006). Eating fast leads to obesity: Findings based on self-administered questionnaires among middle-aged Japanese men and women. *Journal of Epidemiology, 16,* 117–124.

Packard, C. (2009). Nutrition, cognitive wellbeing and socioeconomic status. In C. L. Cooper, J. Field, U. Goswami, R. Jenkins, & B. J. Sahakian (Eds.), *Mental capital and wellbeing.* Malden, MA: Wiley-Blackwell.

Papies, E. K., Stroebe, W., & Aarts, H. (2007). Pleasure in the mind: Restrained eating and spontaneous hedonic thoughts about food. *Journal of Experimental Social Psychology, 43,* 810–817.

Pelchat, M. L. (2009). Food addiction in humans. *Journal of Nutrition, 139,* 620–622.

Petroni, M. L., Villanova, N., Avagnina, S., Fusco, M. A., Fatati, G., Compare, A., . . . the QUOVADIS Study Group. (2007). Psychological distress in morbid obesity in relation to weight history. *Obesity Surgery, 17,* 391–399.

Philipson, T. J., & Posner, R. A. (1999). *The long-run growth in obesity as a function of technological change* (Working Paper No. 7423). Cambridge, MA: National Bureau of Economic Research.

Pine, K. J., & Fletcher, B. C. (2011). Women's spending behaviour is menstrual cycle sensitive. *Personality and Individual Differences, 50*(1), 74–78.

Pinel, J. P. J., Assanand, S., & Lehman, D. R. (2000). Hunger, eating, and ill health. *American Psychologist, 55*(10), 1105–1116.

Polivy, J. (1998). The effects of behavioral inhibition: Integrating internal cues, cognition, behavior, and affect. *Psychological Inquiry, 9,* 181–204.

Polivy, J., & Herman, C. P. (1985). Dieting and bingeing: A causal analysis. *American Psychologist, 40,* 193–201.

Polivy, J., & Herman, C. P. (1999). Distress and eating: why do dieters overeat? *International Journal of Eating Disorders, 26,* 153–164.

Polivy, J., Herman, C. P., & Coelho, J. S. (2008). Caloric restriction in the presence of attractive food cues: External cues, eating, and weight. *Physiology & Behavior, 94,* 729–733.

Powell, L. M. (2009). Fast food costs and adolescent body mass index: Evidence from panel data. *Journal of Health Economics, 28,* 963–970.

Powell, L. M., Chriqui, J. F., & Chaloupka, F. J. (2009). Associations between state-level soda taxes and adolescent body mass index. *Journal of Adolescent Health, 45,* S57–S63.

Power, M. L., & Schulkin, J. (2009). *The evolution of obesity.* Baltimore, MD: Johns Hopkins University Press.

Powell, L. M., Chriqui, J. F., & Chaloupka, F. J. (2009). Associations between stat-level soda taxes and adolescent body mass index. *Journal of Adolescent Health, 45,* S57–S63.

Puhl, R., & Brownell, K. D. (2001). Bias, discrimination, and obesity. *Obesity Research, 9,* 788–805.

Rachlin, H. (2000). *The science of self-control.* Cambridge, MA: Harvard University Press.

Ramachandran, V. S. (2004). *A brief tour of human consciousness.* New York, NY: Pi Press.

Ramey, V. A. (2009). Time spent in home production in the 20th century United States: New estimates from old data. *Journal of Economic History, 69*(1), 1–47.

Raynor, H. A., & Epstein, L. H. (2001). Dietary variety, energy regulation, and obesity. *Psychological Bulletin, 127,* 325–41.

Read, D., & Van Leeuwen, B. (1998). Predicting hunger: The effects of appetite and delay on choice. *Organizational Behavior and Human Decision Processes, 76,* 189–205.

Rogers, P. J., & Smit, H. J. (2000). Food craving and food "addiction": A critical review of the evidence from a biopsychosocial perspective. *Pharmacology, Biochemistry and Behavior, 66,* 3–14.

Rolls, B. (2005). *The volumetrics eating plan.* New York, NY: HarperCollins.

Rolls, B. J. (1986). Sensory-specific satiety. *Nutrition Review, 44,* 93–101.

Rolls, B. J., Roe, L. S., Halverson, K. H., & Meengs, J. S. (2007). Using a smaller plate did not reduce energy intake at meals. *Appetite, 49,* 652–660.

Rolls, B. J., Rolls, E. T., Rowe, E. A., & Sweeney, K. (1981). Sensory specific satiety in man. *Physiology & Behavior, 27,* 137–142.

Rosen, M. (1989). On randomized controlled trials and lifestyle interventions. *International Journal of Epidemiology, 18,* 993–994.

Rosenbaum, M., Sy, M., Pavlovich, K., Leibel, R. L., & Hirsch, J. (2008). Leptin reverses weight loss-induced changes in regional neural activity responses to visual food stimuli. *Journal of Clinical Investigation, 118*(7), 2583–2591.

Roth, D. A. (1999). *The influence of norms on eating behavior: An impression management approach.* Toronto, ON: University of Toronto Dissertation.

Rothman, A. J. (2000). Toward a theory-based analysis of behavioral maintenance. *Health Psychology, 19*(Suppl.), 64–68.

Rothman, A. J., Baldwin, A., & Hertel, A. (2004). Self-regulation and behavior change: Disentangling behavioral initiation and behavioral maintenance. In K. Vohs & R. Baumeister (Eds.), *The handbook of self-regulation* (pp. 130–148). New York, NY: Guilford Press.

Rothman, A. J., Sheeran, P., & Wood, W. (2009). Reflective and automatic processes in the initiation and maintenance of dietary change. *Annals of Behavioral Medicine, 38*(Suppl. 1), S4–S17.

Rozin P., Dow, S., Moscovitch, M., & Rajaram, S. (1998). What causes humans to begin and end a meal? A role for memory for what has been eaten, as evidenced by a study of multiple meal eating in amnesic patients. *Psychological Science, 9,* 392–396.

Rozin, P., Kabnick, K., Pete, E., Fischler, C., & Shields, C. (2003). The ecology of eating: Smaller portion sizes in France than in the United States help explain the French paradox. *Psychological Science, 5,* 450–454.

Saffer, H., & Dave, D. (2002). Alcohol consumption and alcohol advertising bans. *Applied Economics, 34,* 1325–1334.

Sanfey, A. G., Loewenstein, G., McClure, S. M., & Cohen, J. D. (2006). Neuroeconomics: Cross-currents in research on decision-making. *Trends in Cognitive Sciences, 10*(3), 108–116.

Sanfey, A. G., Rilling, J. K., Aronson, J. A., Nystrom, L. E., & Cohen, J. D. (2003). The neural basis of economic decision-making in the ultimatum game. *Science, 300*(5626), 1755–1758.

Sapolsky, R. (2004). *Why zebras don't get ulcers: A guide to stress, stress-related diseases and coping* (3rd ed.). New York, NY: Holt.

Sanfey, A. G., Loewenstein, G., McClure, S. M., & Cohen, J. D. (2006). Neuroeconomics: cross-currents in research on decision-making. *Trends Cogn Sci, 10*(3), 108–116.

Sayette, M. (2004). Self-regulatory failure and addiction. In R. F. Baumeister & K. D. Vohs (Eds.), *Handbook of self-regulation* (pp. 447–465). New York, NY: Guilford Press.

Schachter, S. (1971). Some extraordinary facts about obese humans and rats. *The American Psychologist, 26,* 129–144.

Scharff, R. L. (2009). Obesity and hyperbolic discounting: Evidence and implications, *Journal of Consumer Policy, 32*(1), 3–21.

Schelling, T. (1984). Self-command in practice, in policy, and in a theory of rational choice. *American Economic Review, 74,* 1–11.

Schmidt, H. (2008). Bonuses as incentives and rewards for health responsibility: A good thing? *Journal of Medicine and Philosophy, 33,* 198–220.

Schousboe, K., Visscher, P. M., Erbas, B., Kyvik, K. O., Hopper, J. L., Henriksen, J. E.,… Sorensen, T. I. A. (2004). Twin study of genetic and environmental influences on adult body size, shape, and composition. *International Journal of Obesity, 28,* 39–48.

Schwartz, B. (2004). *The paradox of choice: Why more is less.* New York, NY: Harper Collins.

Schwartz, M. B., Vartanian, L. R., Nosek, B. A., & Brownell, K. D. (2006). The influence of one's own body weight on implicit and explicit anti-fat bias. *Obesity, 14,* 440–447.

Schwarz, N., & Clore, G. L. (1988). How do i feel about it? The informative function of mood. In K. Fiedler & J. Forgas (Eds.), *Affect, cognition and social behavior* (pp. 44–62). Toronto, ON: C. J. Hogrefe.

Shapiro, J. M. (2005). Is there a daily discount rate? Evidence from the food stamp nutrition cycle. *Journal of Public Economics, 89*(2–3), 303–325.

Shapouri, S., & Rosen, S. (2008, July). Global diet composition: Factors behind the changes and implications of the new trends. In *Food Security Assessment, 2007* (GFA-19). Washington, DC: USDA, Economic Research Service. Retrieved from www.ers.usda.gov/publications/gfa19/

Shepard, R. N. (1990). *Mind sights: Original visual illusions, ambiguities, and other anomalies.* New York, NY: WH Freeman and Company.

Shiv, B., & Fedorikhin, A. (1999). Heart and mind in conflict: Interplay of affect and cognition in consumer decision making. *Journal of Consumer Research, 26,* 278–282.

Simon, H. A. (1955). A behavioral model of rational choice. *Quarterly Journal of Economics, 69,* 99–188.

Sirois, F. M. (2004). Procrastination and intentions to perform health behaviors: The role of self-efficacy and the consideration of future consequences. *Personality and Individual Differences, 37,* 115–128.

Sirois, F. M., Melia-Gordon, M. L., & Pschyl, T. A. (2003). "I'll look after my health, later": An investigation of procrastination and health. *Personality and Individual Differences, 37,* 1167–1184.

Small, D. A., Loewenstein, G., & Slovic, P. (2007). Sympathy and callousness: The impact of deliberative thought on donations to identifiable and statistical victims. *Organizational Behavior and Human Decision Processes, 102*(2), 143–153.

Smith, A. (1977) [1776]. *An inquiry into the nature and causes of the wealth of nations.* Chicago, IL: University of Chicago Press.

Smith, J. P. (1999). Healthy bodies and thick wallets: The dual relation between health and economic status. *Journal of Economic Perspectives, 13*(2), 145–166.

Smith, P. K. (2009). *Obesity among poor Americans: Is public assistance the problem?* Nashville, TN: Vanderbilt University Press.

Smith, P. K., Bogin, B., & Bishai, D. (2005). Are time preference and body mass index associated? Evidence from the National Longitudinal Survey of Youth. *Economics and Human Biology, 3,* 259–270.

Sobal, J., & Stunkard, A. J. (1989). Socioeconomic status and obesity: A review of the literature. *Psychological Bulletin, 105,* 260–275.

Södersten, P., Bergh, C., & Zandian, M. (2006). Understanding eating disorders. *Hormones and Behaviour, 50,* 572–578.

Solomon, R. L. (1977). An opponent-process theory of acquired motivation: The affective dynamics of addiction. In J. Maser & M. Seligman (Eds.), *Psychopathology: Experimental models* (pp. 66–103). San Francisco, CA: W. H. Freeman.

Solomon, R. L., & Corbit, J. D. (1973). An opponent-process theory of motivation: 11. Cigarette addiction. *Journal of Abnormal Psychology, 81,* 158–171.

Squires, S. (2005, July 26). Successful losers. *Washington Post,* HE01.

Stanovich, K. E. (2004). *The robot's rebellion: Finding meaning the age of Darwin.* Chicago, IL: Chicago University Press.

Steele, K. E., Prokopowicz, G. P., Schweitzer, M. A., Magunsuon, T. H., Lidor, A. O., Kuwabawa, H., . . . Wong, D. F. (2009). Alterations of central dopamine receptors before and after gastric bypass surgery. *Obesity Surgery, 20*(3), 369–374.

Steele, P. (2007). The nature of procrastination: A meta-analytic and theoretical review of quintessential self-regulatory failure. *Psychological Bulletin, 133*(1), 65–94.

Stice, E., Spoor, S., Ng, J., & Zald, D. H. (2009). Relation of obesity to consummatory and anticipatory food reward. *Physiology & Behavior, 97*(5), 551–560.

Stice, E., Yokum, S., Blum, K., & Bohon, C. (2010). Weight gain is associated with reduced striatal response to palatable food. *The Journal of Neuroscience, 30*(39), 13105–13109.

Stringhini, S., Sabia, S., Shipley, M., Brunner, E., Nabi, H., Kivimaki, M., . . . Singh-Manoux, A. (2010). Association of socioeconomic position with health behaviors and mortality. *The Journal of the American Medical Association, 303*(12), 1159–1166.

Stroebe, W. (2008). *Dieting, overweight, and obesity: Self-regulation in a food-rich environment.* Washington, DC: American Psychological Association.

Ströhle, A., (2009). Physical activity, exercise, depression and anxiety disorders. *Journal of Neural Transmission, 116,* 777–784.

Sturm, R. (2002). The effects of obesity, smoking, and drinking on medical problems and costs. *Health Affairs, 21*(2), 245–253.

Sturm, R., & Datar, A. (2008). Food prices and weight gain during elementary school: 5-year update. *Public Health, 122*(11), 1140–1143.

Stutzer, A. (2007). *Limited self-control, obesity and the loss of happiness* (IZA Discussion Papers 2925). Bonn, Germany: Institute for the Study of Labor (IZA).

Svaldi, J., Brand, M., & Tuschen-Caffier, B. (2010). Decision-making impairments in women with binge eating disorder. *Appetite, 54,* 84–92.

Syed, M. (2010a). *Bounce.* New York, NY: HarperCollins.

Syed, M. (2010b). *Bounce Intl: Mozart, Federer, Picasso, Beckham, and the science of success.* New York, NY: HarperCollins.

Thaler, R. H., & Shefrin, H. M. (1981). An economic theory of self-control. *Journal of Political Economy, 89,* 392–406.

Thaler, R. H., & Sunstein, C. R. (2008). *Nudge: Improving decisions about health, wealth, and happiness.* New Haven, CT: Yale University Press.

Thomas, J. G., & Wing, R. R. (2009). *Maintenance of long-term weight loss.* Retrieved from http://www.rimed.org/medhealthri/2009-02/2009-02-53.pdf

Thorpe, K. E., Florence, C. S., Howard, D. H., & Joski, P. (2004). The impact of obesity on rising medical spending. *Health Affairs, 23*(Suppl. 2), W4-480–W4-486. Retrieved from SCOPUS database.

Tice, D. M., Baumeister, R. F., Shmueli, D., & Muraven, M. (2007). Replenishing the self: Effects of positive affect on performance and persistence following ego depletion. *Journal of Experimental Social Psychology, 43*(3), 379–384.

Tomiyama, A. J., Mann, T., & Comer, L. (2009). Triggers of eating in everyday life. *Appetite, 52,* 72–82.

Tosini, N. (2008). *The socioeconomic determinants and consequences of women's body mass.* Dissertations available from ProQuest. Paper AAI3328665. Retrieved from http://repository.upenn.edu/dissertations/AAI3328665

Ubel, P. A. (2009). *Free market madness: why human nature is at odds with economics— And why it matters.* Boston, MA: Harvard Business Press.

U.S. Department of Agriculture. (2010). *National nutrient database for standard reference.* Retrieved from www.nal.usda.gov/fnic/foodcomp/search

van Strien, T., Herman, C. P., & Verheijden, M. W. (2009). Eating style, overeating, and overweight in a representative Dutch sample: Does external eating play a role? *Appetite, 52,* 380–387.

Verdejo-García, A., López-Torrecillas, F., Giménez, C. O., & Pérez-García, M. (2004). Clinical implications and methodological challenges in the study of the neuropsychological correlates of cannabis, stimulant, and opioids abuse. *Neuropsychology Review, 14*(1), 1–41.

Volpp, K. G., John, L. K., Troxel, A. B., Norton, L., Fassbender, J., & Loewenstein, G. (2008). Financial incentive-based approaches for weight loss: A randomized trial. *Journal of the American Medical Association, 300*(22), 2631–2637.

Vohs, K. D., Baumeister, R. F., & Loewenstein, G. (2007). *Do emotions help or hurt decision making?* New York, NY: Russell Sage Foundation.

Vohs, K. D., & Faber, R. J. (2007). Spent resources: Self-regulatory resource availability affects impulse buying. *Journal of Consumer Research, 33,* 537–547.

Vohs, K. D., & Heatherton, T. F. (2000). Self-regulatory failure: A resource-depletion approach. *Psychological Science, 11,* 249–254.

Volkow, N. D., Wang, G.-J., Fowler, J. S., & Telang, F. (2008). Overlapping neuronal circuits in addiction and obesity: Evidence of systems pathology. *Philosophical Transactions of the Royal Society of London. Series B, Biological Sciences, 363,* 3191–3200.

Volkow, N. D., & Wise, R. A. (2005). How can drug addiction help us understand obesity? *Nature Neuroscience, 8,* 555–560.

Von Ranson, K., & Robinson, K. E. (2006). Who is providing what type of psychotherapy to eating disorder clients? A survey. *International Journal of Eating Disorders, 39*(1), 27–34.

Waber, R. L., Shiv, B., Carmon, Z., & Ariely, D. (2008). Commercial features of placebo and therapeutic efficacy. *Journal of the American Medical Association, 299*(9), 1016–1017.

Wang, G. J., Volkow, N. D., Logan, J., Pappas, N. R., Wong, C. T., Zhu, W., . . . Fowler, J. S. (2001). Brain dopamine and obesity. *Lancet, 357*(9253), 354–357.

Wansink, B. (2006). *Mindless eating: Why we eat more than we think.* New York, NY: Bantham Dell.

Wansink, B., Just, D. R., & Payne, C. R. (2009). Mindless eating and health heuristics for the irrational. *American Economic Review, 99*(2), 165–169.

Wardle, J. (2007). Eating behaviour and obesity. *Obesity Reviews, 8*(Suppl. 1), 73–75.

Weijzen, P. L., de Graaf, C., & Dijksterhuis, G. B. (2008). Discrepancy between snack choice intentions and behavior. *Journal of Nutrition Education and Behavior, 40*(5), 311.

Weller, R. E., Cook, E. W., Avsar, K. B., & Cox, J. E. (2008). Obese women show greater delay discounting than healthy-weight women. *Appetite, 51,* 563–569.

Wertenbroch, K. (1998). Consumption self-control by rationing purchase quantities of virtue and vice. *Marketing Science, 17,* 317–337.

Whiteside, U., Chen, E., Neighbors, C., Hunter, D., Lo, T., & Larimer, M. (2007). Difficulties regulating emotions: Do binge eaters have fewer strategies to modulate and tolerate negative affect? *Eating Behaviors, 8,* 162–169.

Wilkinson, R. G. (1996). *Unhealthy societies: The afflictions of inequality.* London, UK: Routledge.

Wilson, M., & Daly, M. (2003). Do pretty women inspire men to discount the future? *Biology Letters, S4,* 177–179.

Wilson, T. D. (2002). *Strangers to ourselves: Discovering the adaptive unconscious.* Cambridge, MA: Harvard University Press.

Wilson, T. D., & Gilbert, D. T. (2005). Affective forecasting: Knowing what to want. *Current Directions in Psychological Science, 14,* 131–134.

Wing, R. R., & Phelan, S. (2005). Successful weight loss maintenance. *American Journal of Clinical Nutrition, 82*(1, Suppl.), 222S–225S.

Wood, W., & Neal, D. T. (2007). A new look at habits and the habit-goal interface. *Psychological Review, 14,* 843–863.

Wood, W., & Neal, D. T. (2009). The habitual consumer. *Journal of Consumer Psychology, 19,* 579–592.

Wright, R. (1994). *The moral animal: The new science of evolutionary psychology.* New York, NY: Random House.

Yeomans, M. R., Tepper, B. J., Rietzschel, J., & Prescott, J. (2007). Human hedonic responses to sweetness: Role of taste genetics and anatomy. *Physiology and Behavior, 91*(2–3), 264–273.

Yoon, J. H., Higgins, S. T., Heil, S. H., Sugarbaker, R. J., Thomas, C. S., & Badger, G. J. (2007). Delay discounting predicts postpartum relapse to cigarette smoking among pregnant women. *Experimental and Clinical Psychopharmacology, 15,* 176–186.

Zabelina, D. L., Robinson, M. D., & Anicha, C. L. (2007). The psychological tradeoffs of self-control: A multi-method investigation. *Personality and Individual Differences, 43,* 463–473.

Zajonc, R. B. (1965). Social facilitation. *Science, 149,* 269–274.

Index

a-process, in opponent-process model, 157

Abused substances, 151–152

Addiction, 103
bulimia nervosa/binge eating disorders, patients with, 140
cravings, 139
defining, 136
desire to reduce/quit consuming certain foods, 140
giving up other important activities, 140–141
high-calorie consumption, 140
loss of control, 137–138
relapse, 139–140
tolerance, 138
12-step treatment for, 190
withdrawal, 138–139

Affect and cognition, interplay of, 124, 126–127
collaboration and competition, 126

Affect regulation, 167

Affective model, 120–122, 125

Alcohol consumption, 153, 154

Alcohol myopia, 179

"Allostatic load," 86

American Psychiatric Association, 147

Anorexia nervosa, 143, 144–145

Antabuse (disulfiram), 194

Appetitive system, for food consumption, 23

Attentional bias, 165–167

Automatic priming, 127

Automatic self-control, 192
counteractive-control strategy, 203
implementation strategy (if→do rules), 202–203

b-process, in opponent-process model, 157

Bacon, Francis, 198

"Barker hypothesis," 88

Basal metabolic rate, 14

BED. *See* Binge eating disorders (BED)

Behavioral economics, 6, 36, 38, 208
and eating decisions, 1, 5–7
food choice, determinants of, 2–4
multidisciplinary approach, 4–5
neuroeconomics, 37–38
policy implications, 8–9

Binge eating disorders (BED), 136, 137, 141, 146–147, 167, 169

Biological programming, 16, 88

Bitter-taste aversion, 21

"Black box," brain as, 38

Blood sugar, 130

BMI. *See* Body Mass Index (BMI)

Body Mass Index (BMI), 12–13

"Bounded rationality," 37

Brain as "black box," 38

Brain, pleasure center, 151–153
conditioned learning, 152
dopamine, 152–153
reward and motivation system, 152

Bulimia nervosa, 137, 145–146

Buprenorphine, 193

CCK. *See* Cholecystokinin (CCK)

CBT. *See* Cognitive behavioral therapy (CBT)

CHD. *See* Coronary heart disease (CHD)

Childhood obesity, 64

Choice architecture, 208–209

Cholecystokinin (CCK), 17

Cigarette smoking, 62